Healing Is Yours

*Sanctified and cleansed by the
washing of water with the Word*

Paraphrased from Ephesians 5:26

by Patricia L. Whipp

All scripture quotations, unless otherwise indicated, are taken from the New King James Version®. Copyright © 1982 by Thomas Nelson, Inc. Used by permission. All rights reserved.

Healing Is Yours
Copyright © 2013 Patricia L. Whipp

ISBN 10: 0-9723069-5-1
ISBN 13: 978-0-9723069-5-9

All rights reserved. No part of this book may be copied without written permission of the publisher.

The Printed Word
PO Box 7734
La Verne, CA 91750

My child, pay attention to my words,
Incline your ear to my sayings
Do not let them depart from your eyes,
Keep them in the midst of your heart
For they are life to those who find them,
And health to all their flesh.

Proverbs 4:20-22 paraphrased

Healing Is Yours

Reviews

The following reviews have been submitted on this book. The work these people have done to submit these pages is greatly appreciated, and I believe these will be informative for all readers.

From: Carl E. Conley

In 1963, after having been hospitalized many times, I was diagnosed as having an incurable disease. The steps I went through in receiving my complete and total healing all those years ago are clearly laid out in Patricia's book.

In writing this book, Patricia Whipp has provided a valuable service to the body of Christ. While many scholarly treatises have been written on the subject, Patricia has captured the essence of the message. She has brought it to us in clear and understandable language. It is easy to read, clear in its presentation, and organized to enable the reader to appropriate the message.

The scripture portions provided will be a great resource for those who are walking the walk of faith for their healing. I highly recommend this book for those who want to understand and appropriate the healing provided for us in the atonement.

Carl E. Conley, JD, MTH

> Faith Community Churches International
> PO Box 69305
> Tucson, AZ 85737
>
> Website: www.fcciweb.com

From: Tom Barkey

I have found reading Patricia Whipp's book *"Healing Is Yours"* to be quite refreshing. It has brought me back to the basic understanding of healing and the price that Jesus paid for all of us to be well. In fact, at the time I was reading Patricia's book, I received divine healing of a sore throat and fever that I had been suffering for a couple of days. I highly recommend this book to you, not just as a book to read, but a book to keep close by whenever you might face the need to be refreshed on God's wonderful grace of healing.

Tom Barkey, Ph.D.
Senior Pastor, Church of Grace

> Church of Grace
> 22653 Old Canal Road
> Yorba Linda CA 92887
>
> Website: www.churchofgrace.com

From: Louise Brock

As I sat and read I was so impressed by the work that Patricia Whipp has put into this book. She has underlined every thought with the Word of God. Then she has put major and minor sickness and disease in neatly organized categories so that whatever the reader may be dealing with it is so easy to find and use. That is a blessing.

I highly recommend this book to every believer. You need to have this in your library. It is a treasure house of scriptures that you can find and use as you minister to the sick. Pastors, there are many sermons on healing just waiting to be preached and the outlines are right in this book.

It teaches the individual with sickness

how to stand on the Word for personal healing as well as the believers who want to minister to the sick, how to use the scriptures to pray the healing prayers for those being ministered to. This book encourages the sick and the well how to watch the confessions of our mouth, so important to get and to keep our healing.

My heart-felt thanks to Patricia Whipp for this new book and I appreciate her faithfulness to the Father for writing it.

Pastor Dr. Louise Brock
Senior Pastor of Faith Community Church East

> Faith Community Church East
> 8455 E Golf Links Road
> Tucson, AZ 85730-1224
>
> Website: www.fcceast.org
> Website: www.lbrockministries.com

From: Laurie Vervaecke

Patricia states, "Healing has been promised and is available." Throughout this book, Patricia asks many provoking questions:

Do you question that the Bible promises you healing? Do you know anyone, very good Christians included, who has not been sick? Who has not suffered from disease? Are you going to believe the Bible, or are you going to believe the doctor's report? Are you going to trust God despite what you see? Patricia does not leave these and other questions hanging. Patricia points you to the answers found within the Word of God, "The Bible is like medicine for you."

Rev Dr Laurie Vervaecke; Ordained Minister,
    Doctorate Clinical Christian Counseling

Vice President, Global Leadership Network;
President,
    Childhelp Wasatch Front Utah Chapter

Author of: Woman—Why Are You Weeping—
    Abuse the Road to Recovery

Also, a child protection manual for churches:
    Treasure Our Children—
        Create Safe Churches

If interested in training or book purchase:
    ResoluteIM@aol.com

Healing Is Yours

Appreciation

This book has been a very interesting project. It was started in 2011—I had the total outline for the book that year. The first chapter, *Healing is Yours,* was written as a teaching in 2011, and the title of the book was settled then.

The second chapter, *Healing is Mine,* was written in 2012. That teaching was greatly expanded in the book. I had expected to finish the book that year. However, finishing up paper work and other details with the death of my mother delayed the book until 2013. In January, God told me to get this finished before I did anything else.

I have never had so much assistance as has been provided on this book. My sister, Dorothy Webster, has always been a very major help over the years. She does all proofreading and helps with final details of anything I publish. Also, my niece, Joy Reyes, has always been available for proofreading and help.

There have been six other people doing work on this book. Jan Kriz and Rya Hackman both proofread the book. As all of the suggestions came in, Dorothy organized the suggestions that I didn't immediately use and summarized the information for me. Further changes were made from all of those suggestions.

This book has a large selection of scriptures for body parts and diseases. There is also an index with diseases listed and suggestions for category selection. Corinne Loomis and Minerva Glass have checked the cross-reference sections and pointed out mistakes. My nephew's wife, Daniella Webster, is an RN. Her knowledge enabled her to check these lists for medical accuracy. She also had major suggestions of items to add, both diseases and scriptures.

My cousin, Caroline Bryan, checked the scriptures, mainly in the teaching area. She caught some errors and improved the footnotes with her work. Beth Parker obtained reprint information for me. The New King James is stored in poetry style, and I did not want to print scriptures in poetry style. Beth found out what could be done and pointed me to where I could see examples of what I should do.

Lorna Juarez has been my encourager. Almost every week she has had a word of encouragement to keep me moving toward accomplishing this task.

Around the beginning of 2012, a prayer team was formed. People were contacted for prayer for both my ministry and the Printed Word. I was blessed with the number and quality of people who signed up to pray for me when requested. The main thing on their list this spring has been this book.

A **BIG thank you** to each and every one of you.

Table of Contents

Teachings

1. Healing Is Yours   5
2. Healing Is Mine   15
3. Receiving/Maintaining Your Healing   29
4. Reaching for Divine Health   41

Scriptures

6. Healing—General   57
7. Healing—Specific Areas   63

Appendix

8. Healing—Methods   149
9. Meditation   153
10. Index—Cross Reference   155
11. Salvation Information   165
12. Where to Find More Scriptures   169
13. Where to Obtain Scripture Cards   171

Healing Is Yours

Teachings

Healing Is Yours

Healing Is Mine

Receiving/Maintaining Your Healing

Reaching for Divine Health

Healing Is Yours

Healing Is Yours

Healing has been promised in the Bible. It belongs to you. Healing has been promised and is available. There are many places throughout the Bible where God tells you about healing, ways to obtain healing. God wants the best for you.

When Jesus died on the cross, His body was sacrificed for your life today.[1] The stripes from when He was flogged are for your healing.[2] If you are suffering from sickness and disease, you are suffering something for which payment has already been made.

In the Old Testament, we are told that ALL sickness and disease are under the curse of the law. Many specific diseases are listed, but there is one verse which says that any sickness or disease not listed is also included in the curse.[3] In the

---

[1] John 10:10 Jesus came that you might have life abundantly
[2] Isaiah 53:5 With His stripes we are healed
[3] Deuteronomy 28:61 Any disease or sickness not listed is under the curse

New Testament, we learn that you are redeemed from the curse of the law.[4] You also find that you are healed by His stripes.[5]

Do you question that the Bible promises you healing? Do you know anyone, very good Christians included, who has not been sick or who has not suffered from a disease?

Certainly, I do not know anyone who fits this description. At times, I feel that I have had more than my share of opportunities for sickness. However, I continue to stand on the Word. I also continue to see healing in my body.

Make a decision

What do you do? The first step is to make a decision. God said that you must choose life or death. He also told you what to do. He said to choose life![6]

What are you deciding? You can say that you are choosing life, but you need to make a

---

[4] Galatians 3:13 You are redeemed from the curse of the law
[5] 1 Peter 2:24 You are healed by His stripes
[6] Deuteronomy 30:19 Life or death are set before you

more basic decision. What you need to do is to take a look at the Bible, look at healing scriptures, and decide if you are going to believe the Bible, or if you are going to believe what you see. Are you going to believe the Bible, or are you going to believe the doctor's report? Are you going to trust God, despite what you see?

What you see and what the doctor tells you are real. This is how you describe your condition in terms of the world's thinking. They are real; they are facts. What the doctor warns you will happen will occur if you don't do certain things. If he tells you there is no way you will continue to live, you will probably die. These are the facts about which you have to make a decision.

There is a higher way to live

There is a higher truth than the world's facts. There is a higher way to live: that is God and His love for you. God is offering you healing. It is there, available for you. Understand that if you wait too long to make the choice, there may not be time enough for the healing. Many people wait until things are too serious to decide that they need to trust God. Yes, God does miracles, but it's easier to obtain your healing before it reaches that stage. Once you make the decision that you are going to trust God, you will need to take certain steps and hold your ground. That is in chapter three.

Actually, if you start setting your faith before you get sick, it is a lot easier and quicker to obtain a healing. That is in chapter four.

God wants you healed

One thing that needs to be done is to learn, so that it is settled in your mind, that God is not teaching you a lesson, that you don't have the sickness because God wants you sick, or that you have done something which would cause God to not want you healed. Throughout the Bible, it is shown that God has healing for you. He wants you blessed! Nowhere does it say that sickness is a blessing. To think that there could be a good reason for sickness doesn't even make sense!

It is so easy to think you have caused the problem! However, maybe you did cause the problem! Maybe you tried the polar bear swim in January, and ended up with the flu. You might have ridden a motorized scooter too fast, fallen, and broke your collar bone. What about the person who climbed a ladder without being sure that it was secure, fell, and damaged his knee? Repent, apologize to God for not using wisdom, then receive your healing. When God forgives, He forgets, so you are once again eligible to be healed.[7]

God's Word is medicine

Did you know that the Word of God has healing in it? The Word is like medicine for you. If this is a new concept to you, take several scriptures and meditate on them to build this into your soul and into your spirit. This is food for your spirit.

As a suggestion, use the three scriptures on the next page to meditate:

---

[7] Luke 5:20-23 Man forgiven of sins and healed

> Exodus 23:25
> So you shall serve the Lord your God, and He will bless your bread and your water. And I will take sickness away from the midst of you.
>
> Psalm 107:20
> He sent His Word, and healed them, and delivered them from their destructions.
>
> Proverbs 3:8
> It *[The Word]*[8] will be health to your flesh, and strength to your bones.

Read these three scriptures out loud to yourself several times a day. Read them at least five times each time that you do this. Study them. Visualize the time they were first said as they were told to the prophets. As you do this, you are feeding them into your spirit, and you are "renewing" your mind. You are replacing the negative thoughts with these truths.

Have you noticed, God has always provided healing for man? Healing was available under the law; healing was available for all who would believe and trust God. The scriptures listed above are all in the Old Testament. They were available

---

[8] Words in italics added for understanding

before Jesus was crucified. Yes, there is a much better covenant under the New Testament. Obtaining healing may be easier today than it was under the law, but it was and is available.

A mistake that many people make is assuming that they know how they will receive their healing. In the Old Testament, God sent one man[9] to a river to dip seven times before he would receive his healing. If you read that event in the Bible, you will see he did not want to do that. However, his servant suggested to him that he do what the prophet said. As he finished, he was totally healed.

Not all healings take place the same way

In the New Testament, there was a blind man. Jesus spat on the dirt and made mud with the saliva. He then put it on the blind man's eyes. Jesus told the blind man to go to the river and wash the clay off of his eyes. After he did this, he could see![10]

---
[9] 2 Kings 5:9-11 Naaman was told to go dip in the river seven times
[10] John 9:6 Jesus spat and made mud

Those were two very unusual requests. You do not see either of these repeated, but in each case God wanted obedience from the person before they received healing. This is seen today at times in healing meetings. Someone will be told to run, or will be hit, something unusual. However, in each of these cases, the person is healed.

Do expect healing, but don't be concerned if you do not receive it the way you expect. Continue with the doctor unless you are told otherwise. God may use that doctor for your healing; but, if you have a witness to do something different, do it. Don't just decide that you are going to stop medicine, treatment, or whatever is happening, until you know you are supposed to do something different.

If you are seeking God, doing the best that you know to hear Him and to follow His instructions, do not worry about making a mistake. If you make a mistake, He will help you to see what needs to be done.

Don't feel you can't take an aspirin or other medications. God often uses those to help you as you receive your healing.

Some people do not believe that God heals today. They are blinded to the healings taking place around them. There is so much healing going on. One person recently was in a hospital for several weeks. She asked the nurses to tell her about the healings they had witnessed on that ward. They had many stories to tell her.

God heals today

The Bible does not say that healings will end; it gives no ending to God working miracles. There are things which God has said will never happen again. He told us that the earth would never again be flooded. He gave us the rainbow as a sign of this.[11]

If God were to do something as drastic as end healing, or end miracles, don't you think He would have put it in the Bible? There is no indication that these scriptures are not for today. If you need healing, seek God and receive your healing from Him.

---

[11] Genesis 9:12-13 The rainbow is a sign that the earth will never again be flooded

Healing Is Mine

Have you ever gone to a doctor and had him give you a prescription? I expect that most people have had this experience. Then, did you go to the pharmacy and have the prescription filled? After you filled the prescription, did you use it? If it was a salve, did you apply it according to the directions? If it was pills, did you take them as the doctor said to do?

These are very standard steps which most people would follow. What if you brought the medication home, set it on a dresser, in the kitchen, or some other place, and never used it—you never followed any of the directions? Then, you would find that there was no benefit from having paid for this medication!

Do you realize that this is exactly what many people do with healings from God? Many people realize that God heals. They know that God has provided healing for them, that His Son was beaten for their healing, every stripe of the whip provided for their healing.[1] Yet, do you know of people who say they have not received their healing? What they do is ignore the directions to receive their healing. It is very likely that they will not receive their healing. The Bible has very clear instructions about how to receive healing! The directions need to be followed.

When is healing received

One of the first things to learn is when a healing is received. Once again, there are facts about things which happen on this earth. People can look at events, and what they see are "facts." For example, if you have a fever and spots on your body, these are facts. The doctor can see them, anyone can see them. But the truth is Isaiah 53:5, "By His stripes you *are* healed."

Do you notice that scripture is present tense? When did that healing take place? That took place on the day that Jesus was crucified. Has Jesus been crucified? Yes. Now, look at

---

[1] Isaiah 53:5 By His stripes you are healed

1 Peter 2:24. It says, "By whose stripes you *were* healed."[2] Do you see the tense in that sentence? That is past tense. You were healed 2,000 years ago! The truth is that you were healed. There may be an enemy of God trying to convince you otherwise, but the **truth** is that you were healed 2,000 years ago.

Watch the words of your mouth

What has to be done about the facts? One of the first things that needs to be done is to watch the words of your mouth. What you say should always line up with the truth. It should always line up with the Word of God. Keep your tense correct in what you speak.

James tells us that a fountain cannot spout both pure and bitter water.[3] Think of salt water. If you had a bottle of pure water and put just a little bit of salt water in it, then it would become salt water. It would be diluted salt water, but it would no longer be pure. The same thing would happen if you were in a pitch black room. Light

---
[2] 1 Peter 2:24 By His stripes you were healed
[3] James 3:11 Pure water and salt water will mix

one match, and it would no longer be pitch black!

What must you do? You need to realize that God has done all He is going to do about your healing. He let His only Son die on the cross. He allowed His only Son to be beaten for your healing. God's part is done.

Don't lie, but watch your words. If you say, "I caught a cold," you just claimed that cold. You told Satan that he has your permission to bring on a bad cold. If you say, "By His stripes I am healed. I believe I am healed, and I am saying so," then you are letting Satan know that this is not your cold, and that you want no part of it.

Let the redeemed say so

Don't mix your confession with polluted words. God says, "Let the redeemed of the Lord say so."[4] You are redeemed from sickness and disease.[5] This is the truth. Say so. Speak what God says, not what the world says.

---

[4] Psalm 107:2 You are redeemed, say so
[5] Galatians 3:13; Deuteronomy 28:61 You are redeemed from the law, from all sickness

Think about this. What would you do if someone brought a box of snakes to your door and tried to hand it to you? Most people would tell that person to take those snakes and get off of their property! That is the same thing you should do about cold symptoms which start to come onto you. Tell those symptoms that you are the redeemed of the Lord and you are saying so. Tell those symptoms to get off of your body.

Speak the Word of God

God does use doctors to heal people; many times your healing will come through a doctor. You will need to give the doctor enough information of the symptoms you are experiencing for him to find the problem. However, watch what you say, and how you say it. What better example of how to speak can you find than God? Tell the doctor the facts, but then be sure to speak the truth as well. When you are lining up your confession with the Word of God, you will be speaking the truth. "By His stripes I am healed." You are lining up with the Word of God, not with the world.

What you have put into your heart (your spirit) is what will come out of your mouth.[6] This is why it is so necessary to watch what you dwell on, think about, and feed on. If you are constantly watching TV shows that are violent, sexual, or use foul language, then that is what you see and hear—and becomes what you will speak.

Do you need healing? Pray for it

To summarize what has been said: first, if you realize you need healing, then pray for it. You have now involved God in your healing. Possibly your prayer was for direction on the next step you will take.

Seek prayer from someone else. If there is a healing anointing present, that is even better! The main reason for this is that when two or more agree, then it will be done.[7] Now, make your decision, do you accept that healing?[8] It is so easy to assume you have accepted it, but it is

---

[6] Matthew 15:18 What you dwell on, you will speak out of your mouth

[7] Matthew 18:19-20 When two or more agree, then things will be accomplished

[8] Deuteronomy 30:19 You have a choice, choose God's way

your choice. As an act of your will, verbalize your choice and say, "I receive."

Now, believe that you have received. Note, belief is not a feeling. You can feel that you haven't received, you can feel like nothing is happening, you can feel lots of things, but don't be moved by your feelings. Only be moved by truth, and the Word of God is truth. The Words which Jesus spoke are spirit, and they are life.[9] Only believe the Words given to you in the Bible.

Now believe that you have received

Don't be moved by what you see. Remember the story of the ten lepers. Ten men had leprosy. Jesus spoke to them and gave them instructions. As they started to follow the directions, all ten were healed. Only one turned back and thanked Jesus. Leprosy is a disease which, as it progresses, will cause body parts to fall off. An ear, a finger, toes—body parts decay and fall off. Only one man was made whole.[10] The one who came back and said, "Thank you," was made whole. The body

---
[9] John 6:63 God's Words are spirit and life to you
[10] Luke 17:11-19 Only one leper was made whole

parts he had lost were restored. Be the one who says, "Thank you."

As an example, think about what you would do if someone tells you they are giving you a new suit. Do you say thank you when they tell you, or do you say, "When I see the new suit I will thank you"? Be the one who says thank you immediately.

Don't doubt; don't be moved by feelings of doubt. Speak to those feelings. Speak what the Bible says. The scriptures tell you that God called those things which be not as though they were.[11] Next, do not be moved by what you see. Do not be impatient. Just believe. Once you have received, then just believe.[12] If it takes 20 years, just believe.

Don't doubt

Be sure you are ready to receive. One time I was working with a pastor who was doing a healing line. I was standing behind the pastor, available

---

[11] Romans 4:17 Call those things which be not as though they were
[12] Ephesians 6:13-14 Having done all to stand, stand therefore

if there was any assistance needed. There was a deaf lady for whom the pastor prayed.

Later, I heard the pastor talking to the interpreter who was with the deaf lady. The pastor knew that the healing anointing had been present for that lady. He asked the interpreter what happened, why wasn't the woman healed? The interpreter explained that the woman had been in a car accident, and that is where she lost her hearing. She received a large settlement for the hearing loss. She was fearful that she would have to give all of the money back if she received her hearing.

Fear can cause you to not receive healing

These thoughts may not be conscious. You might be standing there thinking how nice it will be to hear music again. But if you haven't dealt with the fear of losing the money, the fear can easily cause you to not receive the healing. Check yourself. Pray and ask God to show you if there is anything standing in the way of your receiving your healing.

Do not be moved by your feelings. Satan can play with your feelings. Belief is not a feeling; it is a decision. Once you have seen scriptures telling you that you are promised a healing, once you have made the decision, do not be moved if it is not manifested instantly, only believe.

Do not be moved by feelings

I heard one lady recently give her testimony. She had a baby against tremendous odds. The doctors expected the woman to die. The date the baby was due was close enough that they thought they could save the baby, but they felt the odds were very high that the mother would die. One doctor kept telling her that she was going to die. She lived; both mother and baby are doing fine. The mother, as she gave the testimony, commented that she was glad she didn't understand the seriousness of one complication which arose. If she had understood, it would have been harder to maintain her faith. Personally, I find that sometimes it is better not to listen too closely to all of the world's facts.

If something has caused you to think you made a mistake in some of the things you have done, then let it go and move forward with what you have learned. Learn to flow with God's directions. Do not step into guilt or condemnation over mistakes you have made! The only person who has not made mistakes is Jesus. Everyone has done something wrong in this area. In the body of Christ, each member is learning. We are growing. Hopefully, we each are taking steps to grow, and we are giving our brothers and sisters space to make mistakes and to grow.

Do not step into condemnation over mistakes

A new-born Christian can usually receive healings easily. However, as you grow, as you learn what God has done for you, more is expected of you. If you start recognizing that you have a part to play in your healing, then it should be easier to grow in this area of your life.

Often a non-Christian will receive healing. Pray for a co-worker who has a headache. When the headache disappears, witness to them!

Do not get into condemnation over mistakes you have made.[13] Just consider each mistake a growing step. Pray and ask God to show you what your next step is. There is always a learning curve. Learning to walk in divine health is not like learning to tie a shoe. Once you learn to tie a shoe, you can always tie a shoe. However, once you learn your addition facts, then you have multiplication, fractions, algebra, geometry, trigonometry, calculus, and advanced math. For some people, there is a similar learning curve for healing. You did not learn math in one year; you will not learn everything about healing in one year. Be thrilled that you are learning, no matter where you are on the curve.

Family sicknesses and diseases

Have you, or do you know of someone who says something like, "In my family, the men always die young. Heart disease runs in our family"? It could be heart disease, cancer, tumors,

---

[13] Romans 8:1 There is no condemnation to those in Christ

thin hair, balding. The list is endless! If that is true in your family, that sounds like a curse! Surprise, you are **free** from the curse.[14] You don't need to accept what you have always heard! Since you have heard it all of your life, you will have to spend time renewing your mind and feeding scriptures into your heart to be free of it. **Freedom** is yours. Believe that, stand on it, and don't give up.

Guess what, God never answers a prayer with a "No." Any prayer that God hears, He will do. He does not hear prayers which are not prayed in faith. Seek God, find His desires in the scriptures.[15] Pray according to His Word.

Any prayer God hears will be done

Did you know that if God hears your prayer, then He gives you what you have asked for? It is so wonderful! All you have to do is find His will about your request, and pray His will![16] How do you know what is God's will? Read the

---

[14] Galatians 3:13; Deuteronomy 28:61 You are redeemed from the law, from all sickness
[15] Psalm 66:18; Matthew 6:7 Wrong thoughts, God does not hear
[16] Mark 11:23; 1 John 5:14-15 Believe what you say, it will be done

Bible! All of God's will is written in the Bible! Find at least two or three scriptures which promise you what you are asking for. Put the scriptures in a formal request which you could call a Petition for what you are praying. Next, it would be good to write it down, sign it, and date it. Then read it out loud to God as your prayer for what you are requesting.

Why should you write it down? It is not necessary, but it is a reminder for you. It shows you what is already yours. Having someone agree over the petition with you will strengthen your prayer.[17] You have prayed it. You know what date you prayed it. If Satan tries to challenge it, you have proof that you have prayed it, so you have proof that it is yours.

---

[17] Matthew 18:19-20; 2 Corinthians 13:1 With two or more, it is strengthened

Receiving/Maintaining Your Healing

There are times in your life when you find yourself in need of healing. You might have a cold, maybe you broke a leg, or there is a rash on your chest. If you broke your leg, you would require immediate attention. A rash, a cold, things of this nature are not something you need to address immediately. However, it is best to have an idea of what you are going to do under any circumstance.

Several areas of healing are available to you. What you do will depend on how severe the problem is, what your experiences with similar problems have been, and what you believe. No matter what you decide to do, there are some steps that you should take. The order of these steps, once again, depends on your decisions.

Look for opportunities to add a healing anointing to your faith. You can use scriptures and pray for yourself, ask someone to pray with you, or go to a healing meeting. There are many ways to do this. No matter how it is done, get God involved in your healing.

Get God involved in your healing

If you are at a meeting and there is an invitation for prayer for healing, I suggest you go forward. You do need to follow the instructions. If you have a rash on your arm, and the invitation is for people with heart problems, wait for the appropriate time for prayer. Sometimes you will be told to stay at your seat.

Even if you go to a doctor, you still want to seek God about your healing.

Now, when do you consider yourself healed? When you prayed! Jesus died on the cross for your healing. He took the stripes on His back for your healing.[1] So, technically, you are healed. When do you see it? Sometimes immediately, sometimes there will be a time lapse before you

---

[1] Isaiah 53:5 By His stripes you are healed

see the healing. This is an area that causes many people to look down on healing ministries. Don't lie, but don't try to confuse or upset people. A simple response is, "I believe I am healed."

When you pray, say, "I receive my healing." You must take some steps in this process. If you wait to see the results, that is not accepting what Jesus has done for you. So, as an act of faith, state, "I receive my healing." God calls those things which be not as though they were.[2] You must learn to act like your Father and do what He is teaching you to do.

Do not wait for results, walk in faith

Don't lie. If you have blood dripping from your arm, don't say, "What blood?" You can say, "I believe it is stopped." You can remain silent. This is an area that causes much confusion for people, non-believers as well as many Christians. Keep your words true to what God says, but don't lie about the facts of what people see.

---

[2] Romans 4:17 Call those things which be not as though they were

When you go to a doctor, you need to learn to pray, use scriptures, and set your faith for the doctor to be led by God and know what you need and how to treat you. I had a skin condition in one area on my body that started with an infection. It lasted several years. At times, the doctor had me coming to see him monthly. He tried different creams. I was praying through all of this.

Then, one day the doctor tried a cream that was not intended for this problem, but it worked. Finally, the day came when he said, "I did not think this was possible, but that skin is completely normal." I asked him if he had tried it on other patients. He told me he did try it on another lady; he saw some results, but nothing like the results I received.

Pray over doctors and medications

I tell doctors when something like this happens that it happened because I add prayer to what they tell me to do. I have prayed over any medication I take. I have prayed for the doctor to be led to do what is needed.

Receiving/Maintaining Your Healing

One thing that you need to do is to find scriptures that you will use as you are believing for your healing. These scriptures need to be quoted out loud daily. You are not convincing God, you are not begging God, you are not into works. You are feeding your spirit with the truth. God's Word is truth and life to your spirit.[3] God's Word is also medicine to your flesh.[4]

Once again, how do you receive healing? It is very simple; you say, "I receive."

Can a healing be lost

Have you ever heard of someone being prayed for at a meeting, watched the healing manifest, and then they lose the healing? That happens, or does it? I have heard of it happening. Recently, I learned that a cousin, who died several years ago, had been prayed for and received her healing. Friends took her to a meeting for this healing. The cousin, and her mother with whom she lived, knew nothing about healings. For several days, she talked clearly and walked with

---
[3] John 6:63 The Word is truth and life
[4] Proverbs 4:22 The Word is life, health, medicine to your flesh

no problem. Both things she could not normally do. Then, she "lost" the healing. No one who could have helped them knew anything about her healing. It wasn't until after the girl had died that her mother shared what had happened.

God has an enemy

Did you know that God has an enemy? His name is Satan. Satan will do his best to convince you that you are not healed. Your mind can work against you. If you start doubting that you are healed, you are giving Satan permission to bring all of the symptoms back. He will!

Find scriptures which help you in the area where you are believing for healing. In this book, you will find a list of general healing scriptures; these scriptures tell you that God wants you healed. You will also find a list of scriptures for body parts and diseases. These are very specific.

My suggestion is to pick three to five scriptures. You may combine these scriptures from either section to find what seems right to you. Find scriptures that give you a peace, that seem to say what you want to say. For example, the scriptures below describe your rights, what you have in Jesus, and what you want to see. If you are having problems walking due to a tumor or ulcer, this would be a reasonable combination of scriptures to use:

> Galatians 3:13
> Christ has redeemed us from the curse of the law, having become a curse for us (for it is written, "Cursed is everyone who hangs on a tree")...
>
> Deuteronomy 28:61
> Also every sickness and every plague, which is not written in this Book of the Law, will the Lord bring upon you until you are destroyed.

(Note: This tells us that ALL sicknesses and plagues are under the curse of the law. You have the right to be free of every sickness and plague. You are redeemed from these.)

> Zechariah 10:12
> "So I will strengthen them in the Lord; and they shall walk up and down in His name," says the Lord.

Read these scriptures out loud several times a day. My suggestion is at least morning and night, read them three to five times each. This will build the truth into your mind and into your spirit. As your body hears the truth, it will respond.

Don't quit! I have quoted scriptures for some areas for several years, and I am now seeing the victory. The blood tests are showing the victory. The doctor is finally convinced that I have the victory in this one area!

There was another problem for which I did not go to the doctor. My muscles all started hurting. It hurt to sit, it hurt to lie down. This went on for several weeks. I spoke to my body, I praised God because I love Him, and I told Him that I love Him. I had a few people in agreement with me. That lasted for three to four weeks. I went to the hospital and prayed for someone else. Shortly after that, the problem lifted and has been gone since then.

You have authority over ALL power of the enemy

Satan is an enemy of God. Why would he attack you? Because you are a child of God. That is one way to cause grief for God, by attacking His children. Did you know that you have authority over ALL the power of the enemy?[5] You have authority over all that Satan can do to you.

How do you exercise this authority? How do you tell disease to get off of you, to get away from you? In the name of Jesus. Every knee shall bow to the name of Jesus.[6] Every tongue shall confess that Jesus is Lord. Flu, colds, measles, broken arms, these are all names. Sickness is a name. Satan is a name. Every one of these names must bow and confess that Jesus is Lord. Every one of them must leave you.

Speak to the mountain

Another scripture tells you to speak to the mountain.[7] Maybe your problem is a mountain in your life. A sickness, disease, or body malfunction could all be a mountain. Speak to that mountain and drive it out of your body.

There are times when I have gotten diagnosed just to have a name to speak. In the area

---

[5] Luke 10:19 You have authority over ALL power of the enemy
[6] Philippians 2:10-11 Every knee shall bow, every tongue confess
[7] Mark 11:23 Speak to the mountain and it shall be removed

where I mentioned previously about the muscles hurting, I did not do this. When a doctor tells me all the problems I have and the medications I should take, and the side effects of the medicines, then sometimes pictures build up in my mind that are hard to deal with. I also pray about what I should do. I'll ask, "Is this a time I need to go to the doctor?"

Pray for direction and guidance

Another possibility to consider is, "Have I been misdiagnosed?" One blood test in my normal testing was bad. I was diagnosed and went to a specialist. I was told that I had a particular list of symptoms. I had none of those symptoms. In fact, my list of problems was the list of the opposite blood test results. (I was told a count was low, my list of symptoms was what happens if the count is too high.)

What have I done? I have sought information from other medical testing. The specialist that I saw would not believe me, so I had to go to other people. The results are still changing and my trust is in the Lord.

Do not think that you know exactly how you will be healed. Healings occur in many ways.[8] Naaman was sent to Elisha for healing.[9] Elisha did not even come out to see Naaman. He simply sent a word to Naaman to go dip in the Jordan. Naaman was insulted, and didn't want to do what he was told. His servant reasoned with him, Naaman did what he was told, and he was healed.

Don't let pride stop your healing

Don't let pride stand in the way of your healing. There are prophets today who sometimes tell people to do some unusual things; but when the instructions are given, follow them.

The Bible tells you to think on what is true.[10] Try to always pray, and think on the good. For example, instead of saying, "Please take this cold away from me," say, "I believe that I am well, that my body functions as it was created to function."

---

[8] Appendix - Chapter 7 Methods of Obtaining Your Healing
[9] 2 Kings 5:10-14 The story of Naaman and Elisha
[10] Philippians 4:8 Think on what is true

Work towards looking at the positive, looking at the desired result. Don't dwell on the negative, on the things that are bad. Keep your mind pointed toward the good.

Finally, **don't quit**! God has promised that if you pray believing, He will answer.[11]

---

[11] Mark 11:24 Pray, believe, and you will receive

Reaching for Divine Health

In the world today there are shots. Flu shots, immunizations, and shots for other diseases! Did you know that the Word of God has shots for you? Scripture can be used to protect you from these things. In the book of Deuteronomy, chapter 28, verses 15-68, you will find a long list of curses that are under the law. Galatians 3:13 says, you are redeemed from the curse of the law. You have the right to walk free from everything listed in Deuteronomy 28. Read those verses sometime to see what you are free from.

Just as you can ignore and not take medication the doctor has prescribed, you can ignore and not make use of the scriptures God has given you. In Deuteronomy 28:22, He tells you that you are free from consumption, fever, and inflammation. In Deuteronomy 28:61, you are told that any disease and any sickness not listed is also under the curse of the law. This means that you are redeemed from every sickness and every disease that exists.

Use these three scriptures as a flu shot! Say, out loud, "Father, in Your Word, based on Deuteronomy 28:22, 61, and Galatians 3:13, you tell me that the flu, consumption, fever, and inflammation are all under the curse of the law. You also say that I am redeemed from the curse of the law. In the name of Jesus, I refuse these. I will not accept them, they have no right to me."

Take scripture booster shots regularly

You can take a booster shot daily. Start your morning with a booster shot. There are probably other things in the list that you would like to add to your confession, but this gives you a good start. Plan on reading these actual scriptures periodically.

Have you noticed that several places in this book have referred to the concept of reading, quoting, and using scriptures?[1] That is very

---

[1] Appendix - Chapter 9 Meditation

important. It is a part of renewing your mind[2] to think like God thinks, and it will feed your spirit.[3] There are more benefits as well, but we will focus on these benefits at this time.

Another scripture tells you that you are sanctified and cleansed by the washing of the water by the Word.[4] The word 'sanctified' means to be set apart, to be holy. Could you be sick and be sanctified? That would be a contradiction of terms. So, a part of using scriptures is to be cleansed of sickness.

Let's look at a scripture from Proverbs:

Proverbs 4:20-21
My son, give attention to my Words;
Incline your ear to my sayings.

Do not let them depart from your eyes; keep them in the midst of your heart....

This was written by Solomon to his son. However, the word 'child' can also be used instead of the word 'son.' These scriptures apply to women as well as men. Writing practices in earlier years used the masculine form when

---

[2] Romans 12:2 Renewing your mind
[3] John 6:63 God's Words are life to your spirit
[4] Ephesians 5:26 Sanctified and cleansed by the Word

talking to both men and women.

Look at the beginning, 'give attention' to my Words. How do you 'give attention' to words? You read them, learn them, study them. The next phrase says to 'incline your ear.' If you are alone, how can you do this? You can read them out loud to yourself. If other people are nearby, this can be done softly. Then the scripture says, "Do not let them depart from your eyes." This is an area which is often overlooked today.

Look at key scriptures regularly

First, memorizing scripture is good. Quoting scripture is good. These are things that need to be done more often today. Have scripture on the tip of your tongue, ready to build up someone else, or to build up yourself; also to remind Satan why he is to leave you alone. Keeping these scriptures in front of your eyes is something that God has also told you to do. Scriptures that you quote fairly often should be written somewhere and periodically reviewed. Keep them where your eyes will see them. You might find you dropped or added a word. However, if for no other reason, you need to see these, keep them in front of your eyes, because that is what God has instructed you to do.

Learn to speak the positive instead of the negative; look for the best at all times.[5] If you yell as a child runs out the door, "Don't go into the street," the last words that child heard were, "Go into the street." Try saying, "Stay in the yard," or "Stay on the sidewalk," or at least, "Look before you cross the street." In Proverbs, you are told that a soft answer can turn away strife. Pleasant words are like a honeycomb.[6] Isn't it much nicer to leave a favorable impression than a negative one?

Negative statements can hurt and cause damage

One negative statement can hurt and cause damage[7] that will take many positive words to

---

[5] http://godswordgoingforth.org/?p=201 — This is Positive Word Scriptures

[6] Proverbs 15:1, Proverbs 16:24 A few examples of soft or pleasant words

[7] http://godswordgoingforth.org/?p=351 — This is Negative Word Scriptures

overcome. My sister heard a teaching on this subject, done in a very dramatic way. Shortly after that teaching, her eight year old son started carrying his three month old brother across a tile floor. The boy had been told he was not to walk with the baby, but he did. He fell on the floor on top of the baby. He became very traumatized over what had happened. Normally, she would have screamed at him for his actions, but because of the teaching she had just heard, she was able to minister to him as she and her husband prepared to go to the hospital with the baby.

Can God trust you with your words

Start working on speaking the positive. When the situation comes that is critical, having this habit established will pay off in a big way. The words of your mouth are so important. God created the whole solar system, the earth, fish, and an atom,[8] all with the Words of His mouth. God wants you to do positive things with your mouth. Can He trust you with your words, or are the words of your mouth not trustworthy? Learn

---

[8] Genesis 1:3-26 God said, and it was

to speak with positive words. It also helps if you learn to speak with God's Words.

There could be a whole chapter, possibly a whole book, written on each of the topics that are being covered in this chapter. You are just being given parts of each area you need to work on to follow the road for divine health. You can't start doing everything at once, so pick one area, and start working on that. Then another. Don't drop the first area when you move to the next area. Add to, don't drop one to do another.

Following the road for divine health

Today's world is becoming more and more complex in many ways. The number of ads for prescription medications is amazing. Do these medications really help? Some doctors are telling people that at certain ages they need to take medications just because of their age. If what you hear, or what you are told to do, does not make sense, you might want to consult with another doctor.

More and more options are becoming

available. There are wellness clinics opening up which do consultation and help people in other ways. It used to be taught that a chiropractor was a quack. Today a chiropractor is more widely accepted than they were years ago. I am watching people being healed in many different ways which includes some of these options that are new.

More health options are available today

No matter what you choose to do, pray about it! Next, if you are looking for a clinic, or a new doctor, find people who have had good experiences at those locations. Don't believe everything you hear, but don't be afraid to try something new. Use wisdom and look for guidance from God in the steps that you take.

Many people say, "I don't hear God. What can I do?" As a start, ask yourself if you have peace over taking the steps you are starting to take. No peace, no steps. If there is peace, that is a start, but when you operate out of fear or without peace, that is not God. Watch for your peace.

Scripture tells you several areas that will

hinder your health. Do you judge others? Most of us were taught to do that from a very early age. Do you look at someone and think that must be a person who is no good because they have a tattoo, or because it is a man wearing earrings?[9] You can back your negative thoughts with scripture. However, let's look at these in a different manner. Jesus died for that person just as much as He died for you. If they are Christians, love them. If they are not, be a witness by being friendly to them. Show the love of Jesus to them.

Envy is not good

Do you envy others? Do you see someone with a new car and envy that they can afford a car that is so nice? Do you look at people who are taller, shorter, skinnier, better built, have a better job, can talk better—and envy them? Some things you are envious over might be things you can do something about, but just haven't. Other things are things there is nothing you can do anything about, and you resent that.

---

[9] Matthew 7:1-2; Luke 6:37 If you judge, you will be judged

None of this is doing you any good. Take the steps you need to take to make corrections, and learn to do what you can about things you cannot change. Maybe all you can do is learn to accept something. However, envy is not going to help you. In fact, Proverbs says that envy is rottenness to the bones.[10] Could cancer in the bone be rottenness to the bones? Could fragile bones be rottenness to the bones?

What about bitterness? Can't it be close to envy? Someone who is not as qualified as you are was given a promotion. Why did that person get the job? You have a degree in the subject. You know more than anyone else in the company about that field. It should have been your job. Do you know how much those thoughts will cost you?

Bitterness, envy, wrath — put these away from you

Bitterness, envy, wrath, put these away from you. Do not talk with corrupt words, which those attitudes would cause you to do. If you

---

[10] Proverbs 14:30 Envy is rottenness to the bones

do talk in that manner, you will grieve the Holy Spirit.[11] You want the Holy Spirit to be with you, not grieved. Learn to watch your words and watch your attitudes. Do not step into negativity, into grievous words. If you grieve the Holy Spirit, you will start walking in another spirit and you can only lose.

Bitterness, jealousy, and envy will cause a bitter root to rise up in you, and instead of producing fruit of the Spirit, you will produce bitter fruit in your life.

Unforgiveness hinders prayers

Has someone treated you unfairly? Possibly your boss, your spouse, or a best friend has done something to you and you have been badly hurt. Maybe they told other people something about you that you didn't want known. No matter what has happened, you cannot afford to walk in unforgiveness. You must forgive. This does not mean that you must subject yourself to more of the same treatment, but you must forgive.

---

[11] Ephesians 4:29-31 Put corrupt words away from you, or you will grieve the Holy Spirit

If you do not forgive, your prayers will be hindered. If you don't forgive, God will not forgive you.[12] That's pretty heavy. What do you need to do? Learn to treat other people the way you want to be treated.[13] This means to be kind to others. Do things for others that they like. Learn to get along with other people.

Forgive yourself

What if you have done something that hurt someone else? It could have been done by accident; it could be something which you didn't realize would upset the person. First you apologize to that person, let them know that you regret your actions, and you will do your best to see that it does not happen again. Now, are you through? Have you forgiven yourself? There is no condemnation to those who are in Christ Jesus.[14] You must forgive yourself.

This may sound weird to some people, but there are people who will beat themselves up

---

[12] Matthew 6:14-15 If you don't forgive, God won't forgive you
[13] Luke 6:31 Treat others as you would want to be treated
[14] Romans 8:1 There is no condemnation to those in Christ Jesus

over wrong actions. You do all that you know to do to correct what happened, but then you must forgive yourself. Learn to forget it. Learn from what happened and do not repeat the action.

Most critical to walking in divine health is learning to walk in love. The one commandment which was given in the New Testament is the Love Law. It is crucial that you start walking in love. That is something that you will spend the rest of your life working on. It's not something you do a few times and say, "I have achieved it. I know how to walk in love." No, it is a lifelong process.

Walk in love

As you start walking in love, you are drawing closer to God.[15] You are learning more to walk as Jesus walked. You are learning more about your Father. As you learn more, you draw closer to Him. As you draw closer to Him, He will draw closer to you. God is love.

As you keep God's Word, His love is

---

[15] James 4:8 Draw nigh to God, He will draw nigh to you

perfected in you.[16] If you love one another, God will dwell in you.[17] Never stop, always continue learning more about how to walk in love.

---

[16] 1 John 2:5 Keep His Word, then His love is perfected in you
[17] 1 John 4:12 Love one another, then God will dwell in you

Scriptures

Healing—General

Healing—Specific Areas

Healing Is Yours

Healing — General

The scriptures in this section are all scriptures which can be used for any disease, or any part of the body. They can also be mixed with the scriptures for **Specific Areas** in the next section.

Exodus 23:25
> So you shall serve the Lord your God, and He will bless your bread and your water. And I will take sickness away from the midst of you.

Numbers 23:19
> God is not a man, that He should lie, nor a son of man, that He should repent. Has He said, and will He not do? Or has He spoken, and will He not make it good?

Psalm 30:2
> O Lord my God, I cried out to You, and You healed me.

Psalm 91:10
> No evil shall befall you, nor shall any plague come near your dwelling...

Psalm 91:16
> With long life I will satisfy him, and show him My salvation.

Psalm 103:3
> Who forgives all your iniquities, Who heals all your diseases...

Psalm 107:20
> He sent His Word and healed them, and delivered them from their destructions.

Proverbs 4:22
> For they are life to those who find them, and health to all their flesh.

Proverbs 4:23
> Keep your heart with all diligence, for out of it spring the issues of life.

Proverbs 17:22
> A merry heart does good, like medicine, but a broken spirit dries the bones.

Isaiah 53:4
> Surely He has borne our griefs, and carried our sorrows; yet we esteemed Him stricken, smitten by God, and afflicted.

Isaiah 53:5
> But He was wounded for our transgressions, He was bruised for our iniquities; the chastisement for our peace was upon Him, and by His stripes we are healed.

Jeremiah 17:14
> Heal me, O Lord, and I shall be healed; save me, and I shall be saved, for You are my praise.

Jeremiah 23:29
> "Is not My Word like a fire?" says the Lord, "and like a hammer that breaks the rock in pieces?"

Jeremiah 32:27
> "Behold, I am the Lord, the God of all flesh. Is there anything too hard for Me?..."

Malachi 4:2
> But to you who fear My name The Sun of Righteousness shall arise with healing in His wings; and you shall go out and grow fat like stall-fed calves.

Matthew 8:16
> When evening had come, they brought to Him many who were demon-possessed. And He cast out the spirits with a word, and healed all who were sick...

Matthew 8:17
> That it might be fulfilled which was spoken by Isaiah the prophet, saying: "He Himself took our infirmities and bore our sicknesses."

Matthew 19:26
> But Jesus looked at them and said to them, "With men this is impossible, but with God all things are possible."

Mark 11:23
> For assuredly, I say to you, whoever says to this mountain, 'Be removed and be cast into the sea,' and does not doubt in his heart, but believes that those things he says will be done, he will have whatever he says.

Mark 11:24
> Therefore I say to you, whatever things you ask when you pray, believe that you receive them, and you will have them.

Mark 16:18
> "...They will take up serpents; and if they drink anything deadly, it will by no means hurt them; they will lay hands on the sick, and they will recover."

Galatians 3:13
> Christ has redeemed us from the curse of the law, having become a curse for us (for it is written, "Cursed is everyone who hangs on a tree")...

Healing—General Scriptures

James 5:14

> Is anyone among you sick? Let him call for the elders of the church, and let them pray over him, anointing him with oil in the name of the Lord.

James 5:15

> And the prayer of faith will save the sick, and the Lord will raise him up. And if he has committed sins, he will be forgiven.

James 5:16

> Confess your trespasses to one another, and pray for one another, that you may be healed. The effective, fervent prayer of a righteous man avails much.

1 Peter 2:24

> Who Himself bore our sins in His own body on the tree, that we, having died to sins, might live for righteousness—by whose stripes you were healed.

3 John 2

> Beloved, I pray that you may prosper in all things and be in health, just as your soul prospers.

Healing—Specific Areas

The scriptures on the following pages are each for a specific area. They can be body parts, sickness or disease, emotions, any area pertaining to a person.

There is a page titled **Use V61**. (This refers to the curses of the law, found in Deuteronomy 28. V61 stands for verse 61.) If you cannot find a topic for the item you want to pray over, very possibly this page will be a help.

In Galatians 3:13, it says that Jesus has redeemed you from the curse of the law. There are many items specifically named under the curse of the law, but Deuteronomy 28:61 specifically says that any sickness or disease not listed is included under the curse of the law. So the topic labeled **Use V61** uses these two scriptures. There are also several more **Use Vxx**. These are pages with different specific areas on each one.

Impossible—There is a section of just scriptures saying that God can do the impossible.

The **Healing—General** scriptures that precede this page are also very useful and can be used for most problems. Check these out!

In the **Appendix** section of this book, you will find an **Index—Cross Reference** of the following pages included with a complete list of other suggestions. It gives you a cross reference to help you find the page that might be useful for you.

List of Specific Areas Included

Abdomen
Arthritis
Autism
Back
Blood
Bones
Burns
Cancer
Childbirth
Constipation
Dehydration
Digestion
Dropsy
Ears
Eating Disorders
Eyes
Eyes and Ears
Feet
Fever
Flesh
Hair
Hands
Heart
Hereditary Diseases
Hips
Hypertension
Immune System
Impossible
Infection/Inflammation
Knees
Learning Disabilities

Legs
Loins
Long Life
Maiming Injuries
Malnutrition
Memory
Mind and Soul
Mouth
Neck
Nervousness
Nose
Obesity/Overweight (Negative, Harsh)
Obesity/Overweight (Positive, Gentle)
Oppression/Depression
Pain
Panic Attacks
Paralysis (Palsy)
Parasites
Peace
Phobia (Fear)
Poisoning
Reproductive System
Respiratory System
Resuscitation
Seizures
Shoulder
Sinews
Skin
Sleep Disorders
Snakebite
Speech Disorders
Teeth
Tongue

Underweight
Use Vxx — See list below
Weakness
Wounds

Curses of the law from Deuteronomy 28
(V21 refers to verse 21)

Use V21 (Plague, consumed...)
Use V22 (Consumption, fever, inflammation...)
Use V27 (Boil, tumor, scab, itch)
Use V28 (Madness, blindness, confusion...)
Use V29 (Grope, not prosper, oppressed...)
Use V32 (Children given to another people)
Use V35 (Severe boils)
Use V41 (Your children go into captivity)
Use V59 (Extraordinary, severe, lingering...)
Use V61 (All sickness and disease not named)
Use V65 (No rest, trembling heart...)

Healing—Specific Areas Scriptures

Abdomen

Use suggestions include: Appendix, Belly, Cholera, Diarrhea, Dysentery, Gall Stones, Hernia, Intestines, Liver, Ovary, Stomach

Proverbs 18:20
> A man's stomach shall be satisfied from the fruit of his mouth; from the produce of his lips he shall be filled.

Acts 28:8
> And it happened that the father of Publius lay sick of a fever and dysentery. Paul went in to him and prayed, and he laid his hands on him and healed him.

Proverbs 3:8
> It *[The Word]* will be health to your flesh, and strength to your bones.
> *(Words in italics added for understanding.)*

Job 23:12
> I have not departed from the commandment of His lips; I have treasured the Words of His mouth more than my necessary food.

Also see: Digestion, Immune System, Infection/Inflammation, Malnutrition, Poisoning, Use V22

Arthritis

Use suggestions include: Joints, Psoriasis, Wrist

Mark 3:3, 5
> And He said to the man who had the withered hand, "Step forward."
>
> And when He had looked around at them with anger, being grieved by the hardness of their hearts, He said to the man, "Stretch out your hand." And he stretched it out, and his hand was restored as whole as the other.

Luke 13:11, 13
> And behold, there was a woman who had a spirit of infirmity eighteen years, and was bent over and could in no way raise herself up.
>
> And He laid His hands on her, and immediately she was made straight, and glorified God.

Also see: Pain, Specific parts of the body affected, Use V22

Autism

2 Timothy 1:7
> For God has not given us a spirit of fear, but of power and of love and of a sound mind.

Romans 15:6
> That you may with one mind and one mouth glorify the God and Father of our Lord Jesus Christ.

1 Corinthians 2:16
> For "who has known the mind of the Lord that he may instruct Him?" But we have the mind of Christ.

Psalm 127:3
> Behold, children are a heritage from the Lord, the fruit of the womb is a reward.

Deuteronomy 28:4
> "Blessed shall be the fruit of your body, the produce of your ground and the increase of your herds, the increase of your cattle and the offspring of your flocks...."

Note: This verse is from the blessings of the Lord.

Also see: Impossible, Mind and Soul, Use V32, Use V41

Back

Psalm 145:14
> The Lord upholds all who fall, and raises up all who are bowed down.

Luke 13:11-12
> And behold, there was a woman who had a spirit of infirmity eighteen years, and was bent over and could in no way raise herself up.
>
> But when Jesus saw her, He called her to Him and said to her, "Woman, you are loosed from your infirmity."

Also see: Arthritis, Bones, Neck, Use V59, Use V61

Blood

Use suggestions include: Aids, Anemia, Diabetes, Hemophilia, Hormones, Issue of Blood, Kidneys, Leukemia, Menopause, Menstrual Difficulties, Sickle Cell Anemia, Thyroid, Veins, Virus

Joel 3:21 (KJV)
> For I will cleanse their blood that I have not cleansed: for the Lord dwelleth in Zion.

Ezekiel 16:6
> "And when I passed by you and saw you struggling in your own blood, I said to you in your blood, 'Live!' Yes, I said to you in your blood, 'Live!'..."

Mark 5:29
> Immediately the fountain of her blood was dried up, and she felt in her body that she was healed of the affliction.

Also see: Bones, Immune System, Infection/Inflammation, Use V61

Bones

Use suggestions include: Leukemia, Menstrual Difficulties, Osteoporosis

Proverbs 3:8
> It *[God's Word]* will be health to your flesh, and strength to your bones.
>
> *(Words in italics added for understanding.)*

Isaiah 58:11
> The Lord will guide you continually, and satisfy your soul in drought, and strengthen your bones; you shall be like a watered garden, and like a spring of water, whose waters do not fail.

Psalm 34:20
> He guards all his bones; not one of them is broken.

Acts 3:7
> And he took him by the right hand and lifted him up, and immediately his feet and ankle bones received strength.

Proverbs 15:30
> The light of the eyes rejoices the heart, and a good report makes the bones healthy.

Also see: Blood, Teeth, Use V22

Burns

Isaiah 43:2
> When you pass through the waters, I will be with you; and through the rivers, they shall not overflow you. When you walk through the fire, you shall not be burned, nor shall the flame scorch you.

Daniel 3:27 (KJV)
> And the princes, governors, and captains, and the king's counsellers, being gathered together, saw these men, upon whose bodies the fire had no power, nor was a hair of their head singed, neither were their coats changed, nor the smell of fire had passed on them.

Also see: Flesh

Cancer

Cancer is a disease known by most people. It can be deadly and tragic. There are only a few verses, in a few translations, which use the word cancer. For that reason, no scriptures are given on this page. Proverbs 14:30 says that envy is rottenness to the bones. At least one translation renders that as cancer in the bones.

Because of the number of cancer patients in the world today, I did want to address suggestions for scriptures to use for healing cancer.

Look at the first section of Healing Scriptures. That section, **Healing—General**, is one where most scriptures given could be used for healing of cancer.

If the doctors give a very negative report, then the page labeled **Impossible** in this section would apply.

Scriptures which apply for the body part where the cancer is located could give a vision of that body part healed. That would be a reasonable set of scriptures to use.

More suggestions would include looking at the curses of the law. You have been redeemed from those curses. The suggested curses for cancer are give below.

Also see: Impossible, Peace, Use V27, Use V59, Use V61

Childbirth

Deuteronomy 28:4
>Blessed shall be the fruit of your body, the produce of your ground and the increase of your herds, the increase of your cattle and the offspring of your flocks.

Exodus 1:19
>And the midwives said to Pharaoh, "Because the Hebrew women are not like the Egyptian women; for they are lively and give birth before the midwives come to them."

Exodus 23:26
>No one shall suffer miscarriage or be barren in your land; I will fulfill the number of your days.

1 Timothy 2:15
>Nevertheless she will be saved in childbearing if they continue in faith, love, and holiness, with self-control.

Psalm 113:9
>He grants the barren woman a home, like a joyful mother of children. Praise the Lord!

Constipation

Matthew 15:17
> Do you not yet understand that whatever enters the mouth goes into the stomach and is eliminated?

Mark 7:18-19
> So He said to them, "Are you thus without understanding also? Do you not perceive that whatever enters a man from outside cannot defile him,
>
> because it does not enter his heart but his stomach, and is eliminated, thus purifying all foods?"

Also see: Abdomen, Dehydration, Eating Disorders, Pain

Dehydration

Use suggestions include: Heat Stroke, Sunstroke

Psalm 63:1
> O God, You are my God; early will I seek You; my soul thirsts for You; my flesh longs for you in a dry and thirsty land where there is no water.

Isaiah 41:17
> "The poor and needy seek water, but there is none, their tongues fail for thirst. I, the Lord, will hear them; I, the God of Israel, will not forsake them...."

Isaiah 49:10
> They shall neither hunger nor thirst, neither heat nor sun shall strike them; for He who has mercy on them will lead them, even by the springs of water He will guide them.

John 6:35
> And Jesus said to them, "I am the bread of life. He who comes to Me shall never hunger, and he who believes in Me shall never thirst...."

Also see: Use V61

Digestion

Use suggestions include: Acid Reflex

Psalm 22:26
> The poor shall eat and be satisfied; those who seek Him will praise the Lord. Let your heart live forever!

Matthew 15:17
> Do you not yet understand that whatever enters the mouth goes into the stomach and is eliminated?

Ecclesiastes 3:13
> And also that every man should eat and drink and enjoy the good of all his labor—it is the gift of God.

Also see: Abdomen, Malnutrition, Mouth, Teeth

Dropsy

Use suggestions include: Edema

Luke 14:2, 4
> And behold, there was a certain man before Him who had dropsy.
>
> But they kept silent. And He took him and healed him, and let him go.

Also see: Feet, Legs

Ears

Use suggestions include: Deafness, Dizziness, Tinnitus, Vertigo

Isaiah 50:4
> "The Lord God has given me the tongue of the learned, that I should know how to speak a word in season to him who is weary. He awakens me morning by morning, He awakens my ear to hear as the learned...."

Isaiah 50:5
> The Lord God has opened my ear; and I was not rebellious, nor did I turn away.

Luke 22:51
> But Jesus answered and said, "Permit even this." And He touched his ear and healed him.

Mark 4:9
> And He said to them, "He who has ears to hear, let him hear!"

Mark 4:23
> "...If anyone has ears to hear, let him hear."

Revelation 2:7
> "He who has an ear, let him hear what the Spirit says to the churches...."

Also see: Eyes and Ears, Impossible

Eating Disorders

Use suggestions include: Anorexia, Binge Eating Disorder, Bulimia, Compulsive Overeating

Daniel 1:15
> And at the end of ten days their features appeared better and fatter in flesh than all the young men who ate the portion of the king's delicacies.

1 Corinthians 6:12
> All things are lawful for me, but all things are not helpful. All things are lawful for me, but I will not be brought under the power of any.

1 Corinthians 10:23
> All things are lawful for me, but not all things are helpful; all things are lawful for me, but not all things edify.

Romans 14:17
> For the kingdom of God is not eating and drinking, but righteousness and peace and joy in the Holy Spirit.

Also see: Abdomen, Digestion, Obesity

Eyes

Use suggestions include: Allergies, Blind, Cataracts, Color Blindness, Glaucoma, Keratitis, Pinkeye

Psalm 146:8
> The Lord opens the eyes of the blind; the Lord raises those who are bowed down; the Lord loves the righteous.

Deuteronomy 34:7
> Moses was one hundred and twenty years old when he died. His eyes were not dim nor his natural vigor diminished.

John 9:1,6-7
> Now as Jesus passed by, He saw a man who was blind from birth.
>
> When He had said these things, He spat on the ground and made clay with the saliva; and He anointed the eyes of the blind man with the clay.
>
> And He said to him, "Go, wash in the pool of Siloam" (which is translated, Sent). So he went and washed, and came back seeing.

Also see: Ears and Eyes, Impossible, Infection/Inflammation, Use V28, Use V65

Eyes and Ears

Proverbs 20:12
> The hearing ear and the seeing eye, the Lord has made them both.

Isaiah 32:3
> The eyes of those who see will not be dim, and the ears of those who hear will listen.

Isaiah 35:5
> Then the eyes of the blind shall be opened, and the ears of the deaf shall be unstopped.

Isaiah 29:18
> In that day the deaf shall hear the Words of the book, and the eyes of the blind shall see out of obscurity and out of darkness.

Isaiah 42:18
> "Hear, you deaf; and look, you blind, that you may see...."

Matthew 13:16
> But blessed are your eyes for they see, and your ears for they hear...

Also see: Ears, Eyes, Use V28, Use V61, Use V65

Feet

Use suggestions include: Ankles, Bunion, Corn, Gout, Lameness, Plantar Fasciitis

Psalm 91:12
> In their hands they shall bear you up, lest you dash your foot against a stone.

Psalm 121:3
> He will not allow your foot to be moved; He who keeps you will not slumber.

Proverbs 3:23
> Then you will walk safely in your way, and your foot will not stumble.

Proverbs 3:26
> For the Lord will be your confidence, and will keep your foot from being caught.

Habakkuk 3:19
> The Lord God is my strength; He will make my feet like deer's feet, and He will make me walk on my high hills.

Acts 14:10
> Said with a loud voice, "Stand up straight on your feet!" And he leaped and walked.

Also see: Knees, Legs, Use V35, Use V61

Healing—Specific Areas Scriptures

Fever

Use suggestions include: Heat Stroke, Malaria, Typhoid

Matthew 8:14-15
> Now when Jesus had come into Peter's house, He saw his wife's mother lying sick with a fever.
>
> So He touched her hand, and the fever left her. And she arose and served them.

John 4:52
> Then he inquired of them the hour when he got better. And they said to him, "Yesterday at the seventh hour the fever left him."

Acts 28:8
> And it happened that the father of Publius lay sick of a fever and dysentery. Paul went in to him and prayed, and he laid his hands on him and healed him.

Also see: Infection/Inflammation, Use V22, Use V61

Flesh

Use suggestions include: Acne, Allergies, Boils, Complexion, Connective Tissue, Dandruff, Eczema, Lupus Erythematosus, Ovary, Rosacea, Shingles, Warts

Job 10:11
> Clothe me with skin and flesh, and knit me together with bones and sinews?

Proverbs 4:22
> For they are life to those who find them, and health to all their flesh.

Job 33:25
> His flesh shall be young like a child's, he shall return to the days of his youth.

Daniel 1:15
> And at the end of ten days their features appeared better and fatter in flesh than all the young men who ate the portion of the king's delicacies.

Jeremiah 32:27
> "Behold, I am the Lord, the God of all flesh. Is there anything too hard for Me?..."

Also see: Infection/Inflammation, Sinews, Skin, Use V22, Use V27, Use V61, Wounds

Hair

Use suggestions include: Baldness, Dandruff

1 Kings 1:52
> Then Solomon said, "If he proves himself a worthy man, not one hair of him shall fall to the earth; but if wickedness is found in him, he shall die."

Luke 21:18
> But not a hair of your head shall be lost.

Luke 12:7
> But the very hairs of your head are all numbered. Do not fear therefore; you are of more value than many sparrows.

Acts 27:34
> Therefore I urge you to take nourishment, for this is for your survival, since not a hair will fall from the head of any of you."

Proverbs 16:31
> The silver-haired head is a crown of glory, if it is found in the way of righteousness.

Proverbs 20:29
> The glory of young men is their strength, and the splendor of old men is their gray head.

Hands

Use suggestions include: Arms, Carpal Tunnel, Fingers, Psoriasis, Wrist

Job 4:3
> Surely you have instructed many, and you have strengthened weak hands.

Psalm 144:1
> Blessed be the Lord my Rock, Who trains my hands for war, and my fingers for battle...

Isaiah 35:3
> Strengthen the weak hands, and make firm the feeble knees.

Mark 3:5
> And when He had looked around at them with anger, being grieved by the hardness of their hearts, He said to the man, "Stretch out your hand." And he stretched it out, and his hand was restored as whole as the other.

Hosea 7:15
> Though I disciplined and strengthened their arms, yet they devise evil against Me...

Also see: Arthritis

Heart

Use suggestions include: Chronic Heart Failure, Heart Disease, Stroke

Psalm 73:26
> My flesh and my heart fail; but God is the strength of my heart and my portion forever.

Psalm 147:3
> He heals the brokenhearted and binds up their wounds.

Psalm 27:14
> Wait on the Lord; be of good courage, and He shall strengthen your heart; wait, I say, on the Lord!

Psalm 31:24
> Be of good courage, and He shall strengthen your heart, all you who hope in the Lord.

Also see: Blood, Hypertension, Use V61, Use V65

Hereditary Diseases

Use suggestions include: Cystic Fibrosis, Down Syndrome, Hemophilia, Sickle Cell Anemia

Ezekiel 18:2-3
> "What do you mean when you use this proverb concerning the land of Israel, saying: 'The fathers have eaten sour grapes, and the children's teeth are set on edge'?
>
> "As I live," says the Lord God, "you shall no longer use this proverb in Israel...."

Ezekiel 18:20-21
> "...The soul who sins shall die. The son shall not bear the guilt of the father, nor the father bear the guilt of the son. The righteousness of the righteous shall be upon himself, and the wickedness of the wicked shall be upon himself.
>
> "But if a wicked man turns from all his sins which he has committed, keeps all My statutes, and does what is lawful and right, he shall surely live; he shall not die...."

Deuteronomy 28:4
> "Blessed shall be the fruit of your body, the produce of your ground and the increase of your herds, the increase of your cattle and the offspring of your flocks.

Note: In the last verse you see the blessings concerning your children. Deuteronomy 28:32 says that your children will go into captivity. That is under the curse of the law.

According to Galatians 3:13, you are redeemed from the curse of the law. A heritage disease could be considered a form of captivity. As you can see from the scriptures on the previous page, you and your children are free from all of these curses.

Note: Leukemia is influenced by heritage, but that is not the cause.

Also see: Use V32, Use V41, Use V59

Hips

Use suggestions include: Lameness, Thigh

Song of Solomon 5:15
> His legs are pillars of marble set on bases of fine gold. His countenance is like Lebanon, excellent as the cedars.

Song of Solomon 7:1
> How beautiful are your feet in sandals, O prince's daughter! The curves of your thighs are like jewels, the work of the hands of a skillful workman.

Job 40:16
> See now, his strength is in his hips, and his power is in his stomach muscles.

Also see: Arthritis, Knees, Legs

Hypertension

Isaiah 26:3
> You will keep him in perfect peace, whose mind is stayed on You, because he trusts in You.

Philippians 4:6
> Be anxious for nothing, but in everything by prayer and supplication, with thanksgiving, let your requests be made known to God...

Isaiah 57:19
> "I create the fruit of the lips: Peace, peace to him who is far off and to him who is near," says the Lord, "And I will heal him."

Isaiah 54:10
> For the mountains shall depart and the hills be removed, but My kindness shall not depart from you, nor shall My covenant of peace be removed," says the Lord, who has mercy on you.

Jeremiah 29:11
> For I know the thoughts that I think toward you, says the Lord, thoughts of peace and not of evil, to give you a future and a hope.

Also see: Blood, Heart, Nervousness, Peace

Immune System

Use suggestions include: Aids, Cholera, Diabetes, Leukemia, Lupus Erythematosus, Polio, Rabies, Tetanus, Typhoid, Virus

Psalm 38:11, 15
> My loved ones and my friends stand aloof from my plague, and my relatives stand afar off.
>
> For in You, O Lord, I hope; You will hear, O Lord my God.

Romans 8:2
> For the law of the Spirit of life in Christ Jesus has made me free from the law of sin and death.

Psalm 91:10
> No evil shall befall you, nor shall any plague come near your dwelling...

Also see: Blood, Poisoning

Impossible

Jeremiah 32:27
> "Behold, I am the Lord, the God of all flesh. Is there anything too hard for Me?..."

Matthew 17:20
> So Jesus said to them, "Because of your unbelief; for assuredly, I say to you, if you have faith as a mustard seed, you will say to this mountain, 'Move from here to there,' and it will move; and nothing will be impossible for you...."

Mark 9:23
> Jesus said to him, "If you can believe, all things are possible to him who believes."

Luke 1:37
> "...For with God nothing will be impossible."

Luke 18:27
> But He said, "The things which are impossible with men are possible with God."

John 15:7
> If you abide in Me, and My Words abide in you, you will ask what you desire, and it shall be done for you.

Also see: Use V22, Use V61

Infection/Inflammation

Use suggestions include: Allergies, Asthma, Bronchitis, Cholera, Cold, Connective Tissue, Eczema, Epidemics, Flu, Hepatitis, Keratitis, Kidneys, Lupus Erythematosus, Lyme Disease, Malaria, Neuritis/Neuropathy, Pinkeye, Plague, Pneumonia, Polio, Quinsy/Tonsillitis, Rabies, Sinus Condition, Tetanus, Tonsillitis, Typhoid, Urinary Tract, Virus

Psalm 91:5-10
> You shall not be afraid of the terror by night, nor of the arrow that flies by day,
>
> nor of the pestilence that walks in darkness, nor of the destruction that lays waste at noonday.
>
> A thousand may fall at your side, and ten thousand at your right hand; but it shall not come near you.
>
> Only with your eyes shall you look, and see the reward of the wicked.
>
> Because you have made the Lord, who is my refuge, even the Most High, your dwelling place,

no evil shall befall you, nor shall any plague come near your dwelling...

Job 5:19
> He shall deliver you in six troubles, yes, in seven no evil shall touch you.

Proverbs 12:21
> No grave trouble will overtake the righteous, but the wicked shall be filled with evil.

Luke 10:19
> Behold, I give you the authority to trample on serpents and scorpions, and over all the power of the enemy, and nothing shall by any means hurt you.

Also see: Arthritis, Blood, Fever, Immune System, Impossible, Use V21, Use V22, Use V27, Use V61

Knees

Use suggestions include: Lameness

Job 4:4
> Your words have upheld him who was stumbling, and you have strengthened the feeble knees...

Isaiah 35:3
> Strengthen the weak hands, and make firm the feeble knees.

Hebrews 12:12
> Therefore strengthen the hands which hang down, and the feeble knees...

Also see: Arthritis, Hips, Legs, Use V35

Learning Disabilities

Psalm 119:99
> I have more understanding than all my teachers, for Your testimonies are my meditation.

Psalm 119:100
> I understand more than the ancients, because I keep Your precepts.

1 Corinthians 1:30
> But of Him you are in Christ Jesus, who became for us wisdom from God—and righteousness and sanctification and redemption...

Daniel 1:17
> As for these four young men, God gave them knowledge and skill in all literature and wisdom; and Daniel had understanding in all visions and dreams.

Also see: Memory, Mind and Soul, Nervousness

Legs

Use suggestions include: Lameness, Prostate, Thigh

Isaiah 35:6
> Then the lame shall leap like a deer, and the tongue of the dumb sing. For waters shall burst forth in the wilderness, and streams in the desert.

1 Samuel 2:4
> "The bows of the mighty men are broken, and those who stumbled are girded with strength...."

Zechariah 10:12
> "So I will strengthen them in the Lord, and they shall walk up and down in His name," says the Lord.

Hebrews 12:13
> And make straight paths for your feet, so that what is lame may not be dislocated, but rather be healed.

Psalm 37:23-24
> The steps of a good man are ordered by the Lord, and He delights in his way.
>
> Though he fall, he shall not be utterly cast down; for the Lord upholds him with His hand.

Also see: Arthritis, Hips, Knees, Paralysis, Use V35

Loins

Use suggestions include: Groin, Hernia, Prostate

Proverbs 31:17 (KJV)
> She girdeth her loins with strength, and strengtheneth her arms.

Ephesians 6:14 (KJV)
> Stand therefore, having your loins girt about with truth, and having on the breastplate of righteousness...

Isaiah 11:5
> Righteousness shall be the belt of His loins, and faithfulness the belt of His waist.

Also see: Abdomen, Legs, Reproductive System, Use V27

Long Life

Psalm 103:5
> Who satisfies your mouth with good things, so that your youth is renewed like the eagle.

Isaiah 40:31
> But those who wait on the Lord shall renew their strength; they shall mount up with wings like eagles, they shall run and not be weary, they shall walk and not faint.

Psalm 91:1
> He who dwells in the secret place of the Most High shall abide under the shadow of the Almighty.

Psalm 91:16
> With long life I will satisfy him, and show him My salvation.

Proverbs 3:1-2
> My son, do not forget my law, but let your heart keep my commands;
> For length of days and long life and peace they will add to you.

Exodus 20:12
> Honor your father and your mother, that your days may be long upon the land which the Lord your God is giving you.

Maiming Injuries

Use suggestions include: Crippled, Lameness

Matthew 15:30-31
> Then great multitudes came to Him, having with them the lame, blind, mute, maimed, and many others; and they laid them down at Jesus' feet, and He healed them.
>
> So the multitude marveled when they saw the mute speaking, the maimed made whole, the lame walking, and the blind seeing; and they glorified the God of Israel.

Acts 14:8-10
> And in Lystra a certain man without strength in his feet was sitting, a cripple from his mother's womb, who had never walked.
>
> This man heard Paul speaking. Paul, observing him intently and seeing that he had faith to be healed,
>
> said with a loud voice, "Stand up straight on your feet!" and he leaped and walked...."

Also see: Pain, Wounds

Malnutrition

Use suggestions include: Vitamin Deficiency

Psalm 37:3
> Trust in the Lord, and do good; dwell in the land, and feed on His faithfulness.

Psalm 37:19
> They shall not be ashamed in the evil time, and in the days of famine they shall be satisfied.

Isaiah 1:19
> If you are willing and obedient, you shall eat the good of the land...

Psalm 22:26
> The poor shall eat and be satisfied; those who seek Him will praise the Lord. Let your heart live forever!

Luke 1:53
> He has filled the hungry with good things, and the rich He has sent away empty.

Also see: Abdomen, Underweight, Weakness

Memory

Use suggestions include: Brain

John 14:26
> But the Helper, the Holy Spirit, whom the Father will send in My name, He will teach you all things, and bring to your remembrance all things that I said to you.

Psalm 119:16
> I will delight myself in Your statutes; I will not forget Your Word.

1 John 2:20
> But you have an anointing from the Holy One, and you know all things.

Also see: Mind and Soul

Mind and Soul

Use suggestions include: Alzheimer's, Brain, Dementia, Depression, Mental Health, Stress

Ephesians 4:23
> And be renewed in the spirit of your mind...

Romans 12:2
> And do not be conformed to this world, but be transformed by the renewing of your mind, that you may prove what is that good and acceptable and perfect will of God.

1 Corinthians 2:16
> For "who has known the mind of the Lord that he may instruct Him?" But we have the mind of Christ.

2 Timothy 1:7
> For God has not given us a spirit of fear, but of power and of love and of a sound mind.

Psalm 138:3
> In the day when I cried out, You answered me, and made me bold with strength in my soul.

Also see: Learning Disabilities, Memory, Nervousness, Oppression, Seizures, Use V28, Use V65, Weakness

Mouth

Use suggestions include: Gums, Jaw, Lips, Taste Buds

Psalm 103:5
> Who satisfies your mouth with good things, so that your youth is renewed like the eagle's.

Proverbs 12:19
> The truthful lip shall be established forever, but a lying tongue is but for a moment.

Proverbs 8:6
> Listen, for I will speak of excellent things, and from the opening of my lips will come right things...

Proverbs 8:7
> For my mouth will speak truth; wickedness is an abomination to my lips.

Psalm 51:15
> O Lord, open my lips, and my mouth shall show forth Your praise.

Also see: Digestion, Speech Disorders, Teeth, Tongue, Use V27, Use V61

Neck

Psalm 3:3
> But You, O Lord, are a shield for me, my glory and the One who lifts up my head.

Psalm 27:6
> And now my head shall be lifted up above my enemies all around me; therefore I will offer sacrifices of joy in His tabernacle; I will sing, yes, I will sing praises to the Lord.

Proverbs 29:1
> He who is often rebuked, and hardens his neck, will suddenly be destroyed, and that without remedy.

Also see: Back, Bones, Shoulder, Sinews

Nervousness

Use suggestions include: Anxiety Attacks, Bipolar, Depression, Menstrual Difficulties, PMS, Stress

Philippians 4:6
> Be anxious for nothing, but in everything by prayer and supplication, with thanksgiving, let your requests be made known to God...

Philippians 4:7
> And the peace of God, which surpasses all understanding, will guard your hearts and minds through Christ Jesus.

Colossians 3:15
> And let the peace of God rule in your hearts, to which also you were called in one body; and be thankful.

1 Peter 5:7
> Casting all your care upon Him, for He cares for you.

John 14:27
> Peace I leave with you, My peace I give to you; not as the world gives do I give to you. Let not your heart be troubled, neither let it be afraid.

Also see: Mind and Soul, Oppression, Panic Attacks, Peace, Use V65, Weakness

Nose

Use suggestions include: Allergies, Sinus Infections

Genesis 2:7
> And the Lord God formed man of the dust of the ground, and breathed into his nostrils the breath of life; and man became a living being.

Job 27:3-4
> As long as my breath is in me, and the breath of God in my nostrils,
>
> my lips will not speak wickedness, nor my tongue utter deceit.

Also see: Respiratory System

Obesity/Overweight

(Negative, Harsh Approach)

Psalm 141:3
> Set a guard, O Lord, over my mouth; keep watch over the door of my lips.

Proverbs 13:25
> The righteous eats to the satisfying of his soul, but the stomach of the wicked shall be in want.

Proverbs 23:2-3
> And put a knife to your throat if you are a man given to appetite.
>
> Do not desire his delicacies, for they are deceptive food.

Galatians 6:8
> For he who sows to his flesh will of the flesh reap corruption, but he who sows to the Spirit will of the Spirit reap everlasting life.

1 Peter 2:11 (KJV)
> Dearly beloved, I beseech you as strangers and pilgrims, abstain from fleshly lusts, which war against the soul...

Also see: Eating Disorders

Obesity/Overweight

(Positive, Gentle Approach)

Job 23:12
> I have not departed from the commandment of His lips; I have treasured the Words of His mouth more than my necessary food.

Psalm 119:103
> How sweet are Your Words to my taste, sweeter than honey to my mouth!

Jeremiah 15:16
> Your Words were found, and I ate them, and Your Word was to me the joy and rejoicing of my heart; for I am called by Your name, O Lord God of hosts.

1 Corinthians 6:19
> Or do you not know that your body is the temple of the Holy Spirit who is in you, whom you have from God, and you are not your own?

Romans 14:17
> For the kingdom of God is not eating and drinking, but righteousness and peace and joy in the Holy Spirit.

Oppression/Depression

Use suggestions include: Stress

Isaiah 10:27
> It shall come to pass in that day that his burden will be taken away from your shoulder, and his yoke from your neck, and the yoke will be destroyed because of the anointing oil.

Philippians 4:6
> Be anxious for nothing, but in everything by prayer and supplication, with thanksgiving, let your requests be made known to God...

Psalm 72:4
> He will bring justice to the poor of the people; He will save the children of the needy, and will break in pieces the oppressor.

Luke 10:19
> Behold, I give you the authority to trample on serpents and scorpions, and over all the power of the enemy, and nothing shall by any means hurt you.

Also see: Mind and Soul, Nervousness, Peace, Use V29

Pain

Use suggestions include: Gall Stones, Headache, Menstrual Difficulties, Plantar Fasciitis, Sciatica, Shingles

Isaiah 53:4
> Surely He has borne our griefs and carried our sorrows; yet we esteemed Him stricken, smitten by God, and afflicted.

Acts 2:24
> Whom God raised up, having loosed the pains of death, because it was not possible that He should be held by it.

Hebrews 12:11
> Now no chastening seems to be joyful for the present, but painful; nevertheless, afterward it yields the peaceable fruit of righteousness to those who have been trained by it.

Revelation 21:4
> "...And God will wipe away every tear from their eyes; there shall be no more death, nor sorrow, nor crying. There shall be no more pain, for the former things have passed away."

Panic Attacks

Proverbs 3:25
> Do not be afraid of sudden terror, nor of trouble from the wicked when it comes...

Psalm 91:5
> You shall not be afraid of the terror by night, nor of the arrow that flies by day...

Psalm 116:3, 6
> The pains of death surrounded me, and the pangs of Sheol laid hold of me; I found trouble and sorrow.
>
> The Lord preserves the simple; I was brought low, and He saved me.

Deuteronomy 28:7
> The Lord will cause your enemies who rise against you to be defeated before your face; they shall come out against you one way and flee before you seven ways.

Also see: Peace, Use V28

Paralysis (Palsy)

Use suggestions include: Cerebral Palsy, Lameness, Lou Gehrig's Disease, Multiple Sclerosis, Muscles, Numbness, Parkinson's Disease, Polio

Isaiah 35:6
> Then the lame shall leap like a deer, and the tongue of the dumb sing. For waters shall burst forth in the wilderness, and streams in the desert.

Matthew 15:30
> Then great multitudes came to Him, having with them the lame, blind, mute, maimed, and many others; and they laid them down at Jesus' feet, and He healed them.

Acts 3:6-7
> Then Peter said, "Silver and gold I do not have, but what I do have I give you: In the name of Jesus Christ of Nazareth, rise up and walk."
>
> And he took him by the right hand and lifted him up, and immediately his feet and ankle bones received strength.

Also see: Impossible, Use V61

Parasites

Use suggestions include: Bed Bugs, Giardia, Malaria, Trichomoniasis

Luke 10:19
> Behold, I give you the authority to trample on serpents and scorpions, and over all the power of the enemy, and nothing shall by any means hurt you.

Psalm 91:3
> Surely He shall deliver you from the snare of the fowler and from the perilous pestilence.

Psalm 91:10
> No evil shall befall you, nor shall any plague come near your dwelling...

Also see: Immune System, Use V21

Peace

Philippians 4:7
> And the peace of God, which surpasses all understanding, will guard your hearts and minds through Christ Jesus.

John 14:27
> Peace I leave with you, My peace I give to you; not as the world gives do I give to you. Let not your heart be troubled, neither let it be afraid.

John 16:33
> "...These things I have spoken to you, that in Me you may have peace. In the world you will have tribulation; but be of good cheer, I have overcome the world."

Psalm 29:11
> The Lord will give strength to His people; The Lord will bless His people with peace.

2 Thessalonians 3:16
> Now may the Lord of peace Himself give you peace always in every way. The Lord be with you all.

Phobia (Fear)

2 Timothy 1:7
> For God has not given us a spirit of fear, but of power and of love and of a sound mind.

Deuteronomy 28:7
> "The Lord will cause your enemies who rise against you to be defeated before your face; they shall come out against you one way and flee before you seven ways...."

Psalm 118:6
> The Lord is on my side; I will not fear. What can man do to me?

Isaiah 41:10
> Fear not, for I am with you; be not dismayed, for I am your God. I will strengthen you, yes, I will help you, I will uphold you with My righteous right hand....

Isaiah 54:17
> "...No weapon formed against you shall prosper, and every tongue which rises against you in judgment you shall condemn. This is the heritage of the servants of the Lord, and their righteousness is from Me," says the Lord.

Also see: Nervousness

Poisoning

Mark 16:18
> "...They will take up serpents; and if they drink anything deadly, it will by no means hurt them; they will lay hands on the sick, and they will recover."

Luke 10:19
> Behold, I give you the authority to trample on serpents and scorpions, and over all the power of the enemy, and nothing shall by any means hurt you.

Exodus 23:25
> "So you shall serve the Lord your God, and He will bless your bread and your water. And I will take sickness away from the midst of you...."

Also see: Abdomen, Snakebite, Use V22, Use V61

Reproductive System

Use suggestions include: Barrenness, Breast, Cystic Fibrosis, Hormones, Menstrual Difficulties, Ovary, PMS

Deuteronomy 7:13
>And He will love you and bless you and multiply you; He will also bless the fruit of your womb and the fruit of your land, your grain and your new wine and your oil, the increase of your cattle and the offspring of your flock, in the land of which He swore to your fathers to give you.

Deuteronomy 7:14
>You shall be blessed above all peoples; there shall not be a male or female barren among you or among your livestock.

Psalm 127:3
>Behold, children are a heritage from the Lord, the fruit of the womb is a reward.

Also see: Hereditary Diseases

Respiratory System

Use suggestions include: Allergies, Asthma, Breathing, Bronchitis, COPD, Emphysema, Lungs, Pneumonia, Sinus Conditions

Acts 17:25
> Nor is He worshiped with men's hands, as though He needed anything, since He gives to all life, breath, and all things.

Isaiah 42:5
> Thus says God the Lord, Who created the heavens and stretched them out, Who spread forth the earth and that which comes from it, Who gives breath to the people on it, and spirit to those who walk on it...

Genesis 2:7
> And the Lord God formed man of the dust of the ground, and breathed into his nostrils the breath of life; and man became a living being.

Also see: Nose, Use V61

Resuscitation

Matthew 10:8
> Heal the sick, cleanse the lepers, raise the dead, cast out demons. Freely you have received, freely give.

Luke 8:54-55
> But He put them all outside, took her by the hand and called, saying, "Little girl, arise."
>
> Then her spirit returned, and she arose immediately. And He commanded that she be given something to eat.

Acts 20:9
> And in a window sat a certain young man named Eutychus, who was sinking into a deep sleep. He was overcome by sleep; and as Paul continued speaking, he fell down from the third story and was taken up dead.
>
> But Paul went down, fell on him, and embracing him said, "Do not trouble yourselves, for his life is in him."

Seizures

Use suggestions include: Epilepsy

Mark 9:25-27
> When Jesus saw that the people came running together, He rebuked the unclean spirit, saying to it, "Deaf and dumb spirit, I command you, come out of him and enter him no more!"
>
> Then the spirit cried out, convulsed him greatly, and came out of him. And he became as one dead, so that many said, "He is dead."
>
> But Jesus took him by the hand and lifted him up, and he arose.

Also see: Mind and Soul, Oppression, Use V61

Shoulder

Isaiah 10:27
> It shall come to pass in that day that his burden will be taken away from your shoulder, and his yoke from your neck, and the yoke will be destroyed because of the anointing oil.

Isaiah 9:4
> For You have broken the yoke of his burden and the staff of his shoulder, the rod of his oppressor, as in the day of Midian.

Isaiah 14:25
> That I will break the Assyrian in My land, and on My mountains tread him underfoot. Then his yoke shall be removed from them, and his burden removed from their shoulders.

Also see: Arthritis, Back, Bones, Neck, Sinews

Sinews

Use suggestions include: Connective Tissue, Lupus Erythematosus, Tendons

Ezekiel 37:5
> Thus says the Lord God to these bones: "Surely I will cause breath to enter into you, and you shall live."

Ezekiel 37:6
> "I will put sinews on you and bring flesh upon you, cover you with skin and put breath in you; and you shall live. Then you shall know that I am the Lord."

Also see: Flesh

Skin

Use suggestions include: Allergies, Boils, Complexion, Dandruff, Eczema, Rosacea, Shingles, Warts

Exodus 34:30
> So when Aaron and all the children of Israel saw Moses, behold, the skin of his face shone, and they were afraid to come near him.

2 Samuel 14:25
> Now in all Israel there was no one who was praised as much as Absalom for his good looks. From the sole of his foot to the crown of his head there was no blemish in him.

Job 33:25
> His flesh shall be young like a child's, he shall return to the days of his youth.

Also see: Flesh, Use V27, Use V61

Sleep Disorders

Use suggestions include: Insomnia

Psalm 4:8
> I will both lie down in peace, and sleep; for You alone, O Lord, make me dwell in safety.

Psalm 3:5
> I lay down and slept; I awoke, for the Lord sustained me.

Psalm 127:2
> It is vain for you to rise up early, to sit up late, to eat the bread of sorrows; for so He gives His beloved sleep.

Proverbs 3:24
> When you lie down, you will not be afraid; yes, you will lie down and your sleep will be sweet.

Also see: Nervousness, Use V65

Snakebite

Psalm 91:13
> You shall tread upon the lion and the cobra, the young lion and the serpent you shall trample underfoot.

Acts 28:3, 5
> But when Paul had gathered a bundle of sticks and laid them on the fire, a viper came out because of the heat, and fastened on his hand.
>
> But he shook off the creature into the fire and suffered no harm.

Also see: Poisoning

Speech Disorders

Use suggestions include: Dumbness, Stuttering

Matthew 9:32-33
> As they went out, behold, they brought to Him a man, mute and demon-possessed.
>
> And when the demon was cast out, the mute spoke. And the multitudes marveled, saying, "It was never seen like this in Israel!"

Isaiah 50:4
> "The Lord God has given Me the tongue of the learned, that I should know how to speak a word in season to him who is weary. He awakens me morning by morning, He awakens my ear to hear as the learned...."

Also see: Mouth

Teeth

Song of Solomon 4:2
> Your teeth are like a flock of shorn sheep which have come up from the washing, every one of which bears twins, and none is barren among them.

Proverbs 3:8
> It *[The Word]* will be health to your flesh, and strength to your bones.
>
> *(Words in italics added for understanding.)*
> *(Note: Bones and teeth have the same minerals.)*

Genesis 49:12
> His eyes are darker than wine, and his teeth whiter than milk.

Also see: Bones, Digestion, Mouth

Tongue

Use suggestions include: Taste Buds

Proverbs 12:18
> There is one who speaks like the piercings of a sword, but the tongue of the wise promotes health.

Psalm 34:13
> Keep your tongue from evil, and your lips from speaking deceit.

Psalm 35:28
> And my tongue shall speak of Your righteousness and of Your praise all the day long.

Psalm 119:172
> My tongue shall speak of Your Word, for all Your commandments are righteousness.

Proverbs 18:21
> Death and life are in the power of the tongue, and those who love it will eat its fruit.

Also see: Mouth

Underweight

Use suggestions include: Vitamin Deficiency

Ezekiel 37:5-6
> Thus says the Lord God to these bones: "Surely I will cause breath to enter into you, and you shall live.
>
> I will put sinews on you and bring flesh upon you, cover you with skin and put breath in you; and you shall live. Then you shall know that I am the Lord."...

Also see: Abdomen, Digestion, Malnutrition

Use V21

Deuteronomy 28:21 is a curse of the law.
You are redeemed from the curse of the law.
Always use Galatians 3:13 with a curse of the law.

Deuteronomy 28:21
> The Lord will make the plague cling to you until He has consumed you from the land which you are going to possess.

Galatians 3:13
> Christ has redeemed us from the curse of the law, having become a curse for us (for it is written, "Cursed is everyone who hangs on a tree")...

Also see: Use V61

Use V22

Deuteronomy 28:22 is a curse of the law.
You are redeemed from the curse of the law.
Always use Galatians 3:13 with a curse of the law.

The Hebrew word translated consumption also means wasting disease.

The Hebrew word mildew also means pale. Hence anemia is a possibility.

Deuteronomy 28:22
> The Lord will strike you with consumption, with fever, with inflammation, with severe burning fever, with the sword, with scorching, and with mildew; they shall pursue you until you perish.

Galatians 3:13
> Christ has redeemed us from the curse of the law, having become a curse for us (for it is written, "Cursed is everyone who hangs on a tree")...

Also see: Abdomen, Blood, Fever, Flesh, Immune System, Infection/Inflammation, Poisoning, Use V61

Use V27

Deuteronomy 28:27 is a curse of the law.
You are redeemed from the curse of the law.
Always use Galatians 3:13 with a curse of the law.

In Deuteronomy 28:27, the Hebrew word translated tumors also means thickening of the skin, boils, or hemorrhoids.

These could include many diseases, including sores, etc. of the gums, mouth, and tongue.

The Hebrew word translated scab is also translated festering sores, or scurvy.

Deuteronomy 28:27
> The Lord will strike you with the boils of Egypt, with tumors, with the scab, and with the itch, from which you cannot be healed.

Galatians 3:13
> Christ has redeemed us from the curse of the law, having become a curse for us (for it is written, "Cursed is everyone who hangs on a tree")...

Also see: Flesh, Infection/Inflammation, Specific part of the body, Use V59, Use V61

Use V28

Deuteronomy 28:28 is a curse of the law.
You are redeemed from the curse of the law.
Always use Galatians 3:13 with a curse of the law.

Deuteronomy 28:28
> The Lord will strike you with madness and blindness and confusion of heart.

Galatians 3:13
> Christ has redeemed us from the curse of the law, having become a curse for us (for it is written, "Cursed is everyone who hangs on a tree")...

Also see: Use V61

Use V29

Deuteronomy 28:29 is a curse of the law.
You are redeemed from the curse of the law.
Always use Galatians 3:13 with a curse of the law.

The Hebrew word translated oppressed is also translated abused.

Deuteronomy 28:29
> And you shall grope at noonday, as a blind man gropes in darkness; you shall not prosper in your ways; you shall be only oppressed and plundered continually, and no one shall save you.

Galatians 3:13
> Christ has redeemed us from the curse of the law, having become a curse for us (for it is written, "Cursed is everyone who hangs on a tree")...

Also see: Use V61

Healing—Specific Areas Scriptures

Use V32

Deuteronomy 28:32 is a curse of the law.
You are redeemed from the curse of the law.
Always use Galatians 3:13 with a curse of the law.

Note: Given to another people could mean many things. There are a lot of possibilities for the use of this verse.

Deuteronomy 28:32
> Your sons and your daughters shall be given to another people, and your eyes shall look and fail with longing for them all day long; and there shall be no strength in your hand.

Galatians 3:13
> Christ has redeemed us from the curse of the law, having become a curse for us (for it is written, "Cursed is everyone who hangs on a tree")...

Also see: Use V41, Use V61

Use V35

Deuteronomy 28:35 is a curse of the law.
You are redeemed from the curse of the law.
Always use Galatians 3:13 with a curse of the law.

Deuteronomy 28:35
> The Lord will strike you in the knees and on the legs with severe boils which cannot be healed, and from the sole of your foot to the top of your head.

Galatians 3:13
> Christ has redeemed us from the curse of the law, having become a curse for us (for it is written, "Cursed is everyone who hangs on a tree")...

Also see: Flesh, Infection/Inflammation, Specific part of the body, Use V61

Healing—Specific Areas Scriptures

Use V41

Deuteronomy 28:41 is a curse of the law.
You are redeemed from the curse of the law.
Always use Galatians 3:13 with a curse of the law.

Note: Captivity could be a disease, kidnapped, there are many possibilities for the use of this verse.

Deuteronomy 28:41
> You shall beget sons and daughters, but they shall not be yours; for they shall go into captivity.

Galatians 3:13
> Christ has redeemed us from the curse of the law, having become a curse for us (for it is written, "Cursed is everyone who hangs on a tree")...

Also see: Use V32, Use V61

Use V59

Deuteronomy 28:59 is a curse of the law.
You are redeemed from the curse of the law.
Always use Galatians 3:13 with a curse of the law.

Deuteronomy 28:59
> Then the Lord will bring upon you and your descendants extraordinary plagues—great and prolonged plagues—and serious and prolonged sicknesses.

Galatians 3:13
> Christ has redeemed us from the curse of the law, having become a curse for us (for it is written, "Cursed is everyone who hangs on a tree")...

Also see: Specific part of the body, Use V61

Use V61

Deuteronomy 28:61 is a curse of the law.
You are redeemed from the curse of the law.
Always use Galatians 3:13 with a curse of the law.

Deuteronomy 28:61
> Also every sickness and every plague, which is not written in this Book of the Law, will the Lord bring upon you until you are destroyed.

Galatians 3:13
> Christ has redeemed us from the curse of the law, having become a curse for us (for it is written, "Cursed is everyone who hangs on a tree")...

Also see: Impossible

Use V65

Deuteronomy 28:65 is a curse of the law.
You are redeemed from the curse of the law.
Always use Galatians 3:13 with a curse of the law.

The Hebrew word for trembling also means anxious.

The Hebrew word for anguish also means sorrow or despair.

Deuteronomy 28:65
> And among those nations you shall find no rest, nor shall the sole of your foot have a resting place; but there the Lord will give you a trembling heart, failing eyes, and anguish of soul.

Galatians 3:13
> Christ has redeemed us from the curse of the law, having become a curse for us (for it is written, "Cursed is everyone who hangs on a tree")...

Also see: Use V61

Weakness

Use suggestions include: Fatigue, Heat Stroke, Sunstroke

Joel 3:10
> Beat your plowshares into swords and your pruning hooks into spears; let the weak say, 'I am strong.'

Ephesians 6:10
> Finally, my brethren, be strong in the Lord and in the power of His might.

Philippians 4:13
> I can do all things through Christ who strengthens me.

Isaiah 40:31
> But those who wait on the Lord shall renew their strength; they shall mount up with wings like eagles, they shall run and not be weary, they shall walk and not faint.

Psalm 68:35
> O God, You are more awesome than Your holy places. The God of Israel is He who gives strength and power to His people. Blessed be God!

Also see: Use V61

Wounds

Jeremiah 30:17
> 'For I will restore health to you and heal you of your wounds,' says the Lord, 'Because they called you an outcast saying: "This is Zion; no one seeks her."'

Ezekiel 34:16
> "I will seek what was lost and bring back what was driven away, bind up the broken and strengthen what was sick; but I will destroy the fat and the strong, and feed them in judgment."

Isaiah 53:5
> But He was wounded for our transgressions, He was bruised for our iniquities; the chastisement for our peace was upon Him, and by His stripes we are healed.

Also see: Infection/Inflammation, Pain

Appendix

Methods of Obtaining Healing

Meditation

Index—Cross Reference

Salvation Information

Where to Find More Scriptures

Where to Obtain Scripture Cards

Healing—Methods[1]

The following is copied from BibleNotes on a website which is noted in the footnote below.

ill — sick or indisposed; producing evil or misfortune; calamitous or unfortunate; an ill end; hostile; bad or evil; wicked; ill repute; not proper; rude or unpolished; ill manners; incorrect; not skillful

Exodus 23:25 - He will take sickness away
Psalm 107:20 - He sent His Word and healed us
Psalm 103:2-3 - Bless the Lord, Who heals me
Proverbs 4:20-22 - His Words are life, health, medicine
Proverbs 17:22 - A merry heart doeth good like medicine
Isaiah 53:4-5 - With His stripes we are healed
Matthew 19:26 - With God all things are possible
3 John 1:2 - I pray that you be in health

METHODS OF OBTAINING HEALINGS

1. Faith and reliance in God's Word
    1 Peter 2:24 - By His stripes I was healed

---

[1] http://godswordgoingforth.org/?p=59

Matthew 8:17 - He took my infirmities, sicknesses

Mark 11:23 - Speak to the mountain, it will move

2. Ask and I will do it

John 14:14 - Ask anything in Jesus' name

Matthew 7:7 - Ask and it will be given you

1 John 5:14-15 - Anything we ask, His will to do it

3. Prayer (to Father in Jesus' name)

Mark 11:24 - When you pray, believe, you'll have it

4. Two or three agree

Matthew 18:19 - As touching anything, it will be done

5. Anointing with oil

James 5:14 - In the name of Jesus

Mark 6:13 - They anointed many that were sick

6. Gift of the Holy Spirit

1 Corinthians 12:9 - Given as a gift of the Holy Spirit

7. Laying on of hands

Mark 16:18 - Lay hands on sick, they will recover

8. Communion

1 Corinthians 11:24-32 - By His stripes we were healed

9. Meditation

Proverbs 4:22 – The Word is health, medicine, healing to our flesh

In praying for others, give God the glory for what He does, give Him the worry for what you cannot see.

Healing Is Yours

Meditation[1]

The following is copied from BibleNotes on a website which is noted in the footnote below.

Meditate — to dwell on anything in thought; to cogitate. To contemplate doing; to plan or intend

Always meditate on the solution, never meditate on the problem. (Meditating the problem is worry.)

Strongs[2] 1897 O—to murmur, imagine, meditate, mourn, mutter, roar, speak, study, talk, utter

Strongs 7878 O—ponder, converse (with oneself, and hence aloud), utter, commune, complain, declare, meditate, muse, pray, speak, talk

Strongs 3191 N—revolve in the mind

WHY MEDITATE

1. Directed to
Joshua 1:8 - Meditate day and night
1 Timothy 4:15 - Meditate on these

---

[1] http://godswordgoingforth.org/?p=64

[2] Strongs Concordance — every Greek word, and every Hebrew word has been assigned a number

2. **Confession brings possession (See Words—Yours)**
   a. Builds your faith
      Romans 10:17 - Faith comes by hearing
   b. Feeds your angels
      Psalm 103:20 - They hearken to do God's Word
   c. Plants seeds
      Mark 4:14 - The sower sows the Word

3. **We are sanctified by the Word of God**
   John 17:17 - Sanctify them by thy truth, thy Word

4. **Renews the mind**
   Ephesians 5:26 - Cleansed by the washing of the Word

5. **Puts God in remembrance to His Word**
   Isaiah 43:26 - Do this that we might plead together

6. **Feeds your spirit**
   John 6:63 - Words I speak to you are spirit, life

7. **Health to your body**
   Proverbs 4:22 - Health to all of your flesh

Index — Cross Reference

Abdomen
Acid Reflex — See Digestion
Acne — See Flesh, Skin
Aids — See Blood, Immune System
Allergies — See Eyes, Flesh, Infection/ Inflammation, Nose, Respiratory System, Skin
Alzheimer's — See Mind and Soul
Anemia — See Blood, Use V22
Angina — See Blood, Heart, Hypertension
Ankles — See Feet, Use V61
Anorexia — See Eating Disorders
Anxiety Attacks — See Nervousness, Panic Attacks
Appendix — See Abdomen
Arms — See Hands
Arthritis
Asthma — See Infection/Inflammation, Respiratory System
Autism
Back
Baldness — See Hair
Barrenness — See Reproductive System
Bed Bugs — See Parasites
Belly — See Abdomen
Binge Eating Disorder — See Eating Disorders

Bipolar — See Nervousness
Blind — See Eyes
Blood
Boils — See Flesh, Skin
Bones
Brain — See Memory, Mind and Soul, Use V61
Brain Injury — See Learning Disabilities
Breast — See Reproductive System, Use V27, Use V59
Breathing — See Respiratory System
Bronchitis — See Infection/Inflammation, Respiratory System
Bulimia — See Eating Disorders
Bunion — See Feet
Burns
Cancer
Carpal Tunnel — See Hands
Cataracts — See Eyes
Cerebral Palsy — See Paralysis
Childbirth
Cholera — See Abdomen, Immune System, Infection/Inflammation
Chronic Heart Failure — See Heart
Chronic Sickness — See Use V59
Cirrhosis — See Abdomen
Cold — See Infection/Inflammation
Color Blindness — See Eyes
Complexion — See Flesh, Skin
Compulsive Overeating — See Eating Disorders
Connective Tissue — See Flesh, Infection/Inflammation, Sinews
Constipation
COPD — See Respiratory System

Corn — See Feet
Crippled — See Maiming Injuries
Cystic Fibrosis — See Hereditary Diseases, Reproductive System
Cysts — See Use V27, Use V59
Dandruff — See Flesh, Hair, Skin, Use V27
Deafness — See Ears
Dehydration
Dementia — See Mind and Soul
Depression — See Mind and Soul, Nervousness, Oppression
Diabetes — See Blood, Immune System, Use V61
Diarrhea — See Abdomen
Digestion
Dizziness — See Ears
Down Syndrome — See Hereditary Diseases
Dropsy
Dumbness — See Speech Disorders
Dysentery — See Abdomen
Dyslexia — See Learning Disabilities
Ears
Eating Disorders
Eczema — See Flesh, Infection/Inflammation, Skin
Edema — See Dropsy
Emphysema — See Respiratory System
Epidemics — See Infection/Inflammation
Epilepsy — See Seizures
Eyes
Eyes and Ears
Fatigue — See Weakness
Fear — See Phobia

Feet
Fever
Fingers — See Hands
Flesh
Flu — See Infection/Inflammation
Gall Stones — See Abdomen, Pain
Giardia — See Parasites
Glaucoma — See Eyes
Gout — See Feet
Groin — See Loins
Growths — See Use V27, Use V59
Gums — See Mouth
Hair
Hands
Headache — See Pain
Heart
Heart Disease —See Heart
Heat Stroke — See Dehydration, Fever,
    Weakness
Hemophilia — See Blood, Hereditary Diseases
Hemorrhoids — See Use V27
Hepatitis — See Infection/Inflammation,
    Use V22
Hereditary Diseases
Hernia — See Abdomen, Loins
Hips
Hives — See Infection/Inflammation, Use V61
Hormones — See Blood, Reproductive System,
    Use V61
Hypertension
Immune System
Impossible
Infection/Inflammation

Insanity —See Mind and Soul, Use V28
Insomnia — See Sleep Disorders
Intestines — See Abdomen
Issue of Blood — See Blood
Itch (Rash) — See Infection/Inflammation,
    Use V27
Jaundice — See Use V22
Jaw — See Mouth
Joints — See Arthritis, Specific part of body,
    Use V61
Keratitis — See Eyes, Infection/Inflammation
Kidneys — See Blood, Infection/Inflammation,
    Use V61
Knees
Lameness — See Feet, Hips, Knees, Legs,
    Maiming Injuries, Paralysis
Learning Disabilities
Legs
Leukemia — See Blood, Bones, Cancer,
    Hereditary Diseases, Immune System
Lips — See Mouth
Liver — See Abdomen
Loins
Long Life
Lou Gehrig's Disease — See Paralysis
Lumps — See Use V27, Use V59
Lungs — See Respiratory System
Lupus Erythematosus — See Flesh, Immune
    System, Infection/Inflammation, Sinews
Lyme Disease — See Infection/Inflammation
Lymphoma — See Blood, Cancer
Maiming Injuries

Malaria — See Fever, Infection/Inflammation, Parasites, Use V22
Malnutrition
Memory
Menopause — See Blood
Menstrual Difficulties — See Blood, Bones, Nervousness, Pain, Reproductive System
Mental Health —See Mind and Soul
Mind and Soul
Mouth
Multiple Sclerosis — See Paralysis, Use V61
Muscles — See Paralysis, Specific part of body, Use V61
Neck
Nervous System — See Use V61
Nervousness
Neuritis/Neuropathy — See Infection/Inflammation, Use V61
Nose
Numbness — See Paralysis, Use V61
Obesity/Overweight (Negative, Harsh Approach)
Obesity/Overweight (Positive, Gentle Approach)
Oppression/Depression
Osteoporosis — See Bones
Ovary — See Abdomen, Flesh, Reproductive System
Pain
Palsy — See Paralysis
Panic Attacks
Paralysis (Palsy)
Parasites
Parkinson's Disease — See Paralysis, Use V61
Peace

Index—Cross Reference

Phobia (Fear)
Pinkeye — See Eyes, Infection/Inflammation
Plague — See Infection/Inflammation, Use V21
Plantar Fasciitis — See Feet, Pain
PMS — See Nervousness, Reproductive System
Pneumonia — See Infection/Inflammation,
    Respiratory System
Poisoning
Polio — See Immune System, Infection/
    Inflammation, Paralysis, Use V61
Psoriasis — See Arthritis, Hands
Prostate — See Legs, Loins
Quinsy/Tonsillitis — See Infection/
    Inflammation
Rabies — See Immune System, Infection/
    Inflammation
Rash — See Use V27
Reproductive System
Respiratory System
Resuscitation
Rosacea — See Flesh, Skin
Sciatica — See Pain, Use V61
Scurvy — See Use V27
Seizures
Shingles — See Flesh, Pain, Skin
Shoulder
Sickle Cell Anemia — See Blood, Hereditary
    Diseases, Pain
Sinews
Sinus Conditions — See Abdomen, Digestion,
    Infection/Inflammation, Nose,
    Respiratory System
Skin

Sleep Disorders
Snakebite
Soul — See Mind and Soul
Speech Disorders
Stomach — See Abdomen
Stress — See Mind and Soul, Nervousness,
   Oppression
Stroke — See Heart, Use V59, Use V61
Stuttering — See Speech Disorders
Sunstroke — See Dehydration, Weakness
Taste Buds — See Mouth, Tongue
Teeth
Tendons — See Sinews
Tetanus — See Immune System, Infection/
   Inflammation
Thigh — See Hips, Legs
Thyroid — See Blood, Use V61
Tinnitus (Ringing of the ear) — See Ears
TMJ — See Mouth
Tongue
Tonsillitis — See Infection/Inflammation
Trichomoniasis — See Parasites
Tuberculosis — See Use V22
Tumors — See Use V27, Use V59
Typhoid — See Fever, Immune System,
   Infection/Inflammation
Ulcers — See Specific part of body, Use V27,
   Use V61
Underweight
Urinary Tract — See Infection/Inflammation,
   Use V61
Use Vxx — See list of curses following this
   index

Veins — See Blood, Use V61
Vertigo — See Ears
Virus — See Blood, Immune System, Infection/Inflammation
Vitamin Deficiency — See Malnutrition, Underweight, Use V27
Warts — See Flesh, Skin, Use V27, Use V59
Weakness
Wounds
Wrist — See Arthritis, Hands

Curses of the law from Deuteronomy 28
(V21 stands for verse 21)

Use V21 (Plague, consumed...)
Use V22 (Consumption, fever, inflammation...)
Use V27 (Boil, tumor, scab, itch)
Use V28 (Madness, blindness, confusion...)
Use V29 (Grope, not prosper, oppressed...)
Use V32 (Children given to another people)
Use V35 (Severe boils)
Use V41 (Your children go into captivity)
Use V59 (Extraordinary, severe, lingering...)
Use V61 (All sickness and disease not named)
Use V65 (No rest, trembling heart...)

Salvation Information

Are you born again? Have you made Jesus your Lord and Saviour? If you were to die today, do you know that you would go to heaven?

If you are not sure about any of the above questions, then make Jesus your Lord and Savior. How can you do that? Read the confession in the next two paragraphs out loud.

> **I confess with my mouth that I believe that Jesus is Lord. I believe in my heart that God has raised Jesus from the dead.**
>
> **I receive Jesus as my Lord and Saviour. Thank you God that I now know I am born again.**

The confession which you have just made is taken from the Bible. It is Romans 10:9-10.

Tell someone what you have done. Find a church where people believe in being born again, and where they use and teach the Bible. It is so important to learn what is in the Bible, what God is telling you. It is also good to have fellowship with other people who can help you learn more.

Contact us and let us know that you have now received Jesus as your Lord and Saviour. Contact information is available on the following pages.

Salvation Information

Healing Is Yours

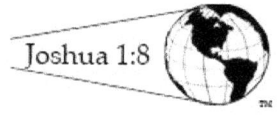

Where to Find More Scriptures

God's Word Going Forth
PO Box 8015
La Verne, CA 91750

Email: Contact@godswordgoingforth.org

Website: godswordgoingforth.org

If you would like to work on other areas of your life besides healing, you can go to the above website. There are over 140 pages of BibleNotes. From these notes, you can find other scriptures. Examples would be:

Anger
Forgiveness
Body of Christ

These would each have different scriptures listed, as well as other useful information.

Did you receive Jesus as your Lord and Saviour on the previous page? Please contact us by email, the website, or a letter to the above address. We look forward to hearing from you.

Healing Is Yours

Where to Obtain Scripture Cards

The Printed Word
PO Box 7734
La Verne CA 91750

Email: CardSets@printedword.org

Website: printedword.org

You can purchase sets of scripture cards on the website listed above. There are 20-60 cards in each set, with a different scripture on each card. Titles include:

>Confidence (Power in Your Words)
>Fear Not
>Wisdom

as well as many more.

Also, at this site you will find books and CDs with scriptures on them. There are scripture card sets in Spanish as well as English.

www.ingramcontent.com/pod-product-compliance
Lightning Source LLC
Chambersburg PA
CBHW070549050426
42450CB00011B/2782